EVERY LIVING CREATURE

EVERY LIVING CREATURE

How Xenotransplantation Will Change Our Lives

JOSHUA D. MEZRICH, MD

The MIT Press
Cambridge, Massachusetts
London, England

The MIT Press
Massachusetts Institute of Technology
77 Massachusetts Avenue
Cambridge, MA 02139
mitpress.mit.edu

The MIT Press would like to thank the anonymous peer reviewers who provided comments on drafts of this book. The generous work of academic experts is essential for establishing the authority and quality of our publications. We acknowledge with gratitude the contributions of these otherwise uncredited readers.

This book was set in Adobe Garamond Pro by New Best-set Typesetters Ltd. Printed and bound in the United States of America.

Library of Congress Cataloging-in-Publication Data is available.

ISBN: 978-0-262-05116-3

10   9   8   7   6   5   4   3   2   1

EU Authorised Representative: Easy Access System Europe, Mustamäe tee 50, 10621 Tallinn, Estonia | Email: gpsr.requests@easproject.com

Contents

Preface

Friday, January 7, 2022. Baltimore, Maryland

Dr. Bartley Griffith was ready to go. The patient was on the operating room (OR) table, their chest split open with a gaping hole where the failing dilated lump of a heart previously was. The patient's life was being sustained by a cardiopulmonary bypass machine. Griffith asked for the new heart, which was carefully removed from its own perfusion circuit, a bypass machine of sorts that was pumping cold oxygenated preservation solution through the organ until it could be placed in its new home.

As Griffith stared at the healthy young heart he was about to sew into his patient, he had a flutter in his own chest. This heart was small, so much smaller than the failing organ he had just removed. Would he be able to fashion the connections of this little heart to the recipient's own blood vessels, and would it be strong enough to give his patient life? The OR was entirely silent except for the quiet hum of the bypass machine, as it temporarily performed the job that this new heart would soon be tasked with.

Everyone in the room understood the enormity of what was about to occur. Griffith had performed more than a thousand human heart transplants in his forty-year career. He was among the most experienced heart transplant surgeons in the world, and even in his early seventies, he was still at the top of his game. But as he looked at this lifeless muscle that he held in his hand, more pale and opaque than any other heart he had ever sewn in, doubt crept into his mind. Maybe this time he was pushing the limits of what was possible just a bit too far.

Griffith took a deep breath and placed the small heart into the massive chest cavity. He asked for his fine suture, roughly the size of a human hair, and began expertly sewing the heart in place. Once he began the stitching, muscle memory took over. All the hesitation and fear (yes, fear, for Griffith is a human just like the rest of us) left his body. The entire team responded to his confidence, his expertise. After Griffith tied the last stitch, and made sure everyone was ready, he released the clamps, allowing his patient's blood to flow into the heart. Suddenly it looked much bigger, much stronger—like it was meant to be in this cavity, this patient. The paleness of the organ was replaced by a healthy pink color. "It was as if we'd turned on a light. And it was a red light. The heart just brightened up. And it went from trembling to pumping. It was one of the best hearts I've ever seen after transplantation."[1]

It was just like any of the other transplants Griffith had performed over his prodigious career. Only it wasn't. Because this heart, twisting and dancing, was tasting human blood for the first time. For this heart, now sustaining life for David Bennet Sr., a fifty-seven-year-old Maryland man, had come from a pig.

* * * * *

In 2020, 7,400 patients in the United States sat waiting for heart transplants, many literally gasping for air while praying for hearts that may never come. Some two hundred died waiting, and a thousand more desperate people were added to the list.[2] The liver transplant waitlist numbered 25,000, and the lung transplant waitlist topped 4,000 patients.[3] In 2020, almost 140,000 patients were waiting for kidneys in the United States, and 24,000 kidney transplants were performed that year. That may sound promising—until one considers that 40,000 new patients were added to the list that same year.[4] Most of these patients spent the year sitting in dialysis chairs three days per week, hooked up to machines with gigantic needles poking into their arms, anxiously waiting for kidneys to become available. That represents more than 175,000 patients who spent their days praying for organs that would have to come from other people's tragedies, if they would come at all.

But these numbers don't begin to capture how many patients in the United States are suffering from end organ damage. The number of patients with end-stage renal disease on dialysis is far higher: just under 600,000. Patients with cirrhosis, or end-stage scarring of the liver, tops 630,000. About 1.5 million people in this country need supplemental oxygen to breathe, many because their lungs are too damaged to perform the way they were designed. Topping the list, an estimated 6 million people suffer from heart failure. The vast majority of these patients will never make it to the transplant list, and likely will never even be referred for evaluation. They are deemed too sick, too old, too alone (you need to have support to get listed), or too poor (you need insurance and a stable housing situation to get a transplant in this country), or they are never even seen by appropriate health care providers who might think of transplant as an option. Even for patients that are deemed "appropriate" and healthy for organ transplant, many die each year waiting for organs that will never come. There will never be enough organs.

Roughly 60 percent of adults in the United States sign up to be organ donors. But less than 1 percent of those people will die in a way that allows for organ donation, which generally requires dying in the hospital with functioning organs. This 1 percent of donors often die from head trauma—typically from a car or motorcycle accident or a gunshot to the head—or from a drug overdose, stroke, or heart attack. In 2020, 12,587 people made up that one percent, donating one or more organs as a deceased donor.

In the end, our patients are stuck in the paradigm that someone has to die in order for someone else to live. There can be another way. Xeno-transplantation, or the transplantation of organs between different species (including from a non-human animal to a human), has been the dream of transplant surgeons since before the first successful allotransplant (between the same species) was performed in 1954. Early attempts transplanting chimpanzee kidneys into humans showed great promise, but insurmount-able challenges related to the fear of a pandemic from a xeno-virus and the protests of animal rights activists—and outcomes not improving fast enough to quell these objections—led to a moratorium on transplanting animal organs into humans in the early 1990s.

As we celebrate the seventieth anniversary of that first successful human allotransplant in 1954, we can reflect on how much has changed in our understanding of science and immunology, and on what might actually be possible when it comes to prolonging life. The field of transplantation itself went from science fiction to clinical reality in a period of thirty years, and since then our ability to rescue people dying from organ failure with human organs has exceeded all expectations. But with this success came unexpected frustration: we will never be able to save the millions of patients that could benefit from transplantation until we find an unlimited source of organs.

Although clinical xenotransplantation faced a moratorium, scientific exploration never stopped. Despite expansion of the armamentarium of powerful medications that can suppress the immune system, it became clear that simply using increasingly potent immunosuppressive drugs would never be enough on its own to allow clinical xenotransplantation to succeed. Something more radical, something transcendent, would be needed. Something like a better understanding of our own biology, of the evolutionary steps that led us to differentiate from other species, and an ability to manipulate those genetic differences in a rapid and reliable way to accelerate particular pathways of evolution in a species that could then serve as compatible donors for humans.

Perhaps as important as any individual scientific discoveries, a new generation of visionaries with the genius to apply these advances; the gravitas to convince patients, clinicians, regulatory bodies, and investors to take this leap; and the hubris to actually think it might work would need to come to the forefront at just the right time.

This book will tell the story of xenotransplantation, beginning with early efforts in the 1960s—when a few promising successes were buried under even more tragic failures—to the disappointments and protestations of the 1980s, which led to a moratorium in the field. It will describe the scientific advances that slowly improved survival in animal models, and then the quantum jumps in our understanding of cloning, gene editing, and infectious disease that have brought us to this particular moment in time. The book will dig deeply into the lives of the modern visionaries who are dedicated to making xenotransplantation a reality no matter the cost, both personal and financial.

This is not just a story of one small discipline of medicine that affects the lives of a few hundred thousand people. It is a story of an innovation so transformative that it will change how we look at what is possible for humankind. It will alter how we look at aging and disease, offering a new paradigm for the prevention of death. In the near future, we will be able to replace any organ using genetically modified bespoke pigs, transplanted electively before a patient suffers any of the effects of an impending disease. Heart disease, renal failure, diabetes, liver failure, and lung disease will all be diseases of the past. It sounds crazy, maybe impossible. But it's not.

I have been thinking about xenotransplantation for twenty-five years. It was 1999, halfway through my surgery training, when I entered a lab in Boston focused on animal models of xenotransplantation. We transplanted hearts and kidneys from genetically modified pigs into monkeys, trying to understand why they would be rejected and what we could do to prolong their survival. Back then, our ability to edit the pigs' genes was rather unsophisticated and painstaking, and it seemed like the experiments would never amount to anything beyond a bunch of presentations, papers, and grants that might advance our academic careers.

Over the next few decades, as I immersed myself in the field of transplantation, I experienced the elation of transplanting life-saving organs into patients facing certain death, watching them recover quickly and completely. The miracle of it is dramatic, truly god-like. As a practicing transplant surgeon, I can tell you that it is a tremendous honor to play a role in the gift of life. And yet, as powerful, uplifting, and even addictive as it is to transplant patients, it is equally devastating to watch patients suffer and die waiting for the gift of life, or to sit at our listing meeting as we decline someone for the transplant list because we know there just aren't enough organs to go around. No matter how hard we try to find organs for our patients, pushing the limits of what organs we will consider adequate for transplantation and educating the public on the importance of being donors, there will never be enough.

However, over the last decade, those of us in the "xeno" community have experienced a growing sense of optimism. A remarkable convergence of advances in gene editing, novel immunosuppressive protocols, and the emergence of a fascinating group of visionaries straight out of central casting has led to a palpable buzz of excitement that I like to term "xeno-optimism." Nearly every month, new records are set in xenotransplant survivals in animal models. Money has poured in from industry and the government to support pre-clinical efforts. Over the last few years, humans have received genetically modified pig hearts and kidneys under compassionate use protocols, and, for the first time ever, human trials with genetically modified pig kidneys are expected to begin in 2025.

A few years ago, I wrote a book about transplantation titled *When Death Becomes Life*.[5] It celebrates the beauty of transplantation, and explains why I consider organ donors to be our patients as much as our recipients are. Our field would not exist without their selfless gifts of life that will forever be their legacies. Despite that, we are nearing a time when we can turn the page on the concept that it takes a death to save a life. It won't happen overnight. It will surely take years, decades maybe. But remember, it only took thirty years to figure out allotransplantation, starting from that first successful transplant in 1954.

I knew this was the perfect time to tell the story of xeno, a true miracle on par with putting a human on the moon. The evocative title *Every Living Creature* captures the idea that all living organisms share similar basic building blocks—DNA—that encode the blueprint for the structure and function of the components that make life possible. Postulating that a primate organ could replace a human organ was a reasonable assumption for early xenotransplant researchers, but the idea that a heart or a kidney from a common farm animal could function in a human was deemed preposterous. It was only by deciphering genetic codes, defining the many similarities and distinct differences between porcine and human genes, and developing a mastery of gene editing and cloning that the seemingly impossible could become a reality. Animals as disparate to us as pigs could be altered, cloned and bred to generate an endless supply of organs for humans. Not long ago, many in our field predicted this was impossible. As the famous surgeon Norm Shumway, known as the father of heart transplantation, stated: "Xenotransplantation is the future of transplantation. And it will always be the future of transplantation."

Welcome to the future.

1 THE PRIMATE ERA BEGINS (1963–1973)

The first successful kidney transplant in humans was performed on December 23, 1954, between identical twins. Over the next decade, a modicum of success was achieved using kidneys from non-identical living and deceased donors. But the outcomes were poor, with greater than 90 percent of those transplants failing, and the recipients dying in a matter of weeks to months. Despite those horrific outcomes, patients with kidney disease had no other hope. Kidney transplant was their only chance for survival, and most patients would give anything to have even a sliver of hope. In this era before brain death was even defined, very few of those patients had access to donors. They were simply going to die. But there was one person who thought it might be possible to try something unconventional to save their lives. That man was Keith Reemtsma, a thirty-eight-year-old surgeon fresh out of training, and that unconventional treatment was xenotransplantation. Despite the dramatic improvement in transplant outcomes over the last seventy years, with better than 95 percent one-year survival in patients today, the longest successful xenotransplant of any organ into a human is still a kidney xenotransplant perfomed by Reemtsma at Charity Hospital in New Orleans in 1964. How did Reemtsma find himself in a situation in which it made sense to transplant chimpanzee kidneys into dying humans, and what gave him the inner confidence that he could accomplish something so revolutionary when so few others were willing to try? This is where the modern story of xeno began.

––––––––––

Keith Reemtsma was born on December 5, 1925 in Madera, California.[1] His father Henry was a Presbyterian minister and missionary. When Reemtsma was thirteen, his family moved to Fort Defiance, Arizona for missionary work on the Navajo Reservation. Fort Defiance was a small government-sponsored post consisting of just 3,900 acres in the 16-million-acre Navajo reservation, where sixty-eight thousand Navajos lived.

As a thirteen-year-old, young Keith Reemtsma enjoyed outdoor activities including horseback riding, and could always be found playing with the Navajo children. But even from a young age, he had a passion for observing the local surgeon working in the operating room. He also enjoyed assisting his parents in the large tuberculosis sanitorium.

Reemtsma entered college at the University of Idaho-Southern Branch with the goal of becoming a doctor. He was so focused that he finished his required pre-medical courses in two years. He entered the University of Pennsylvania School of Medicine in 1945. After an extremely successful four years at medical school, he entered surgery residency at Columbia University College of Physicians and Surgeons in New York City in 1949.

After completing his internship in 1950, Reemtsma found himself in a Mobile Army Surgical Hospital (MASH) unit in Korea, sharing a tent with Frank Spencer, the chief of surgery of the forward marine unit, EZ Medical Company, 1st Medical Battalion, known as the "Cheaters of Death." Spencer, like Reemtsma, grew up in a rural setting in a small town in Texas, and would ultimately become a famous surgeon and chairperson at New York University in New York City. In 1950, after three years of surgical training, he was drafted into military service and sent to Korea. Although the same age as Reemtsma, his three years of training made him the senior surgeon at the unit. It might seem strange to have such inexperienced "surgeons" running MASH units in a war, but that was the policy enacted by the military after World War II, to protect more senior surgeons from having to give up their practices and travel halfway around the world to operate in tents.[2]

These MASH units were extremely busy, treating more than twenty thousand patients each year and performing more than two hundred surgeries per day. Reemtsma arrived in Korea with a footlocker full of scotch, and was known for his wisecracking and for mixing top-notch martinis. He was rumored to have been the inspiration for the character Hawkeye Pierce in the television show *M*A*S*H*, a rumor he did little to contradict.[3] At one point during the run of the hit show, actor Alan Alda actually visited Reemtsma for inspiration for his character, the consummate surgeon who loved pranks and practical jokes. What Reemtsma lacked in experience, he made up for with a larger-than-life personality, confidence, and the ability to find humor in any scenario. When he walked into a room, he immediately owned it.

The war in Korea was a time of massive innovation in surgical care, and Reemtsma was in the thick of it, taking part in numerous novel operations to save the lives and limbs of injured soldiers. Often this meant breaking military rules to perform complex vascular reconstructions, rather than the quicker amputations that the military mandated in their handbooks. But Reemtsma wasn't one to worry about the rules. He always told his trainees to live by the epithet, "It's better to ask for forgiveness than permission." There is little doubt that his experience in Korea, flouting the rules to save lives and limb, risks be damned, played a role in that personal philosophy.

Reemtsma returned from Korea to New York in 1954 and resumed his residency at Columbia. His experience with vascular injuries sparked an interest in bypass surgery, and he developed a particularly keen interest in cardiac surgery (surgery of the heart). This was a new and emerging field, attracting only the most adventurous surgeons. The first successful open-heart surgery using a cardiopulmonary bypass machine was conducted in Philadelphia while Reemtsma was in Korea in May of 1953, and only a few intrepid centers were considering opening their own departments. After completing his training, Reemtsma was recruited to Tulane University in 1957 to build a cardiac surgery service.

Reemtsma arrived in New Orleans ready to do so, a risky endeavor for a newly minted surgeon. When he got there, however, he had nothing to do. Surgeons weren't performing coronary bypass surgeries and valve replacements back then. Reemtsma was hoping to find children who had simple congenital abnormalities in their hearts that needed fixing. But due to difficulty in diagnosis and a lack of specialists in that area, he had to look elsewhere to stay busy. Reemtsma wanted to be busy. But he also wanted to be innovative. If he wasn't going to be able to make his mark in open-heart surgery, he needed to identify another field in its infancy.

Kidney transplantation fit the bill. It was just three years earlier, in 1954, that Joe Murray had performed the first successful kidney transplant in the world, at the Peter Bent Brigham Hospital in Boston, Massachusetts. In 1958, Murray's team at the Brigham began a series of non-identical kidney transplants from living donors with steroids and total body irradiation for immunosuppression. In 1959, he had his first success, with a kidney that lasted 29 years. Still, however, most of the patients would die horrible deaths.[4]

This was the state of the field when Reemtsma entered it in New Orleans in 1957. At the time, he used twins or siblings as donors, treating them with steroids and irradiation. They had minimal access to cadaveric organs for transplant. In the 1950s and 1960s, there was no concept known as "brain death" (it wouldn't be defined until 1968 and wouldn't become equivalent to legal death in the United States until 1981). So in order to have a cadaveric donor, someone relatively healthy would have to die in the hospital at the same time that a recipient happened to be admitted. Preservation solution hadn't yet been invented, so time was of the essence. In Reemtsma's own words, "[w]hen a person dies there is a period of only about one hour in which his kidney can be transplanted to a live person. Often it is impossible to make the complicated preparations in such a short time."[5] The first successful kidney from a cadaver donor wasn't performed until April 5, 1962, again with Joe Murray as the surgeon. So when Reemtsma started in 1957, the only viable donors for transplantation were living donors, and the only viable recipients were those patients that had access to them. To make matters worse, in these early years, dialysis could only be conducted for weeks to months before terminal complications would ensue. Patients without living donors would simply die.

By mid-1963, Reemtsma and his team had performed seven kidney transplants in humans; the first between identical twins had occurred in 1959. But as gratifying as it was to offer those patients at least some chance of survival, in the vast majority of his cases, he couldn't do anything. There was no treatment plan to describe, no options to discuss, no answers for these pleading patients. They had no hope. Death was imminent. That didn't sit well with Reemtsma, a man whose comfort with taking risks and breaking the rules was forged in his hardscrabble upbringing in Fort Defiance and the chaotic years repairing torn limbs and blood vessels in a tent in Korea. Reemtsma was unwilling to tell his patients that he had nothing to offer them, just as he was unwilling to let the limbs of those young soldiers be amputated when he thought he could fix them.

As Reemtsma wrote himself in 1989, "[a] quarter of a century ago I began a study of the use of non-human kidneys transplanted into patients with end-stage renal disease . . . We did not have chronic dialysis, nor did we have cadaveric organs for transplantation. For those reasons we chose to explore non-human donors, and the donors were chimpanzees which had been discarded from circuses and from the space program."[6] It helped that a regional primate facility was established in Louisiana right around this time, allowing for access to primates and experts in primate biology. It's hard to imagine the courage it must have required to embark on a set of experiments like this. Reemtsma was a young surgeon at the beginning of his career, entirely unknown in the field of surgery, already risking his reputation performing kidney transplants at a time when outcomes were horrible and the community at large thought those performing them were crazy. The vast majority of surgeons (me included) would have been too afraid to perform human transplants in that era. The risk was so high, the complication rate astronomical, the likelihood of a miserable death almost expected. The idea that Reemtsma considered it reasonable to transplant *primate* organs into humans says something about the man himself. He would do anything to offer hope to his patients, regardless of the outcomes. He would ask for forgiveness later. He had no fear to embark on a new and risky strategy that clearly seemed outrageous to all of his colleagues. The patients surely thought he was crazy at first, but many were willing to try. When there is no other hope, crazy can seem a lot more normal.

In his first attempt, Reemtsma transplanted two kidneys from a twenty-five-pound male rhesus monkey into a patient that had no potential living donor and no ability to continue dialysis. The operation was reported in the lay press three days after the surgery. The recipient's name and age were withheld, but it was noted that she was a young, married woman. The kidneys worked right away. Reemtsma was very careful in his comments to the press, stating that he could not predict how long the kidneys would last.[7] The kidneys from the rhesus monkey began to fail one week after transplant, and were removed at ten days. In a press release on Saturday, October 19, 1963, it was announced that the kidneys had to be removed due to a loss of function, and that the patient was resting comfortably, in the same condition she was in prior to the xenotransplant. She died the next day. That was always going to be the outcome.

One month later, Reemtsma was attending to another young man with failing kidneys. The patient was a forty-three-year-old dockworker by the name of Jefferson Davis. Davis was diagnosed with high blood pressure in 1957, and a kidney biopsy in 1959 showed significant kidney disease. He was readmitted in June of 1963 with renal failure and was started on temporary dialysis. There was no option for long-term dialysis for Davis, and death was imminent.

In mid-October, amid multiple lengthy conversations discussing Davis's options, Reemtsma first raised the issue of transplantation. He told Davis he could continue supportive therapy, which would mean continued dialysis while in the hospital; ultimately, however, he would be sent home to die. Reemtsma asked Davis if he had a living donor for kidney transplant. Unfortunately, Davis didn't have an identical twin, and although he had a wife and four children, none were appropriate candidates to be living donors. Davis made it clear to Reemtsma that he wanted to live and would do whatever he could to have a chance. As these discussions were ongoing, Reemtsma continued to search for a deceased donor kidney for Davis. But given that the first successful deceased donor kidney had been performed just one year earlier in Boston, Reemtsma was not very optimistic.

Unlike the first xenotransplant in which a rhesus monkey was used, Reemtsma had decided he would next use a chimpanzee as a donor. This was for a number of reasons. First, chimpanzees were known to share a high percentage of genes with humans—somewhere between 96 to 99 percent of DNA. Rhesus monkeys, on the other hand, share roughly 90 percent of DNA with humans. Chimpanzees were also larger, with weights closer to

100 pounds, compared to rhesus monkeys that average closer to 20 pounds. Chimpanzees were also thought to have more efficient kidneys than monkeys. Finally, chimpanzees were known to have blood types A and O (a rare finding in other primates). Because Reemtsma's team had the ability to type the donors prior to transplant, this would increase their odds of finding a blood-type compatible donor for Davis.[8]

"On the morning of November 5, 1963, I went to the operating rooms of Charity Hospital in New Orleans to exchange a few words with my patient, a 43-year-old dock worker in kidney failure. I had spent a long time with him over the past several weeks explaining what I planned to do, and he had agreed. Then I went to Tulane Medical School, next door to Charity Hospital, and shaved a chimpanzee that had been discarded, because of irascibility, by a circus. He had been selected as a donor based on body size and blood group. Then I took the chimpanzee on a journey to Charity Hospital."[9]

Reemtsma and his team wheeled this irascible donor into the operating room next door to Davis, partially shaved and mostly covered in sheets, just like any other patient might be. Reemtsma placed a football helmet on the chimpanzee's head, so the nurses and other patients wouldn't notice his patient was an ape as he wheeled through the corridors of this massive hospital. That was the kind of humorous touch Reemtsma loved, and he would recount the story for years to come. Rumor has it the "sisters" in the OR were quite startled by the very hairy arms in this particular patient, entirely unaware that this donor wasn't a human. Reemtsma wouldn't have bothered to disclose that his donor was a chimpanzee to the OR staff; he would ask for forgiveness later.

Reemtsma performed the donor surgery. He removed both kidneys en bloc, still attached to each other by their blood vessels. At the same time, Davis was put to sleep in the adjoining operating room next door. An incision was made over the right side of his abdomen, and his blood vessels exposed. Once the kidneys were ready for implantation, Reemtsma scrubbed into Davis's operation.

Reemtsma sewed the chimpanzee kidneys into Davis using the same technique we use today. The clamps were removed and the kidneys turned pink, now perfused with Davis's blood—human blood. Within minutes, urine began squirting out of both chimpanzee ureters. The chimpanzee kidneys were without blood for a total time of thirty-nine minutes, a respectable implant time to this day.

Reemtsma then sewed each ureter separately into Davis's bladder and closed him up. In the first fourteen hours after transplantation, the urine output was 6,700 milliliters. That's almost nineteen cans of soda. (A healthy person typically makes one to two liters in twenty-four hours.) His kidney function quickly returned to normal. Davis continued on immunosuppressive drugs that he had started a week before transplant, which included azathioprine, steroids, and a third drug that we no longer use. Four days after the transplant, Davis suffered what was likely a rejection episode—his urine output dropped, he had a fever, and his creatinine went up. His antirejection medications were increased and "X-ray doses" were administered. His urine output and creatinine returned to normal. On the third week postoperatively, Davis had a decline in kidney function and a fever. He received more radiation and his kidneys recovered.[10]

"I feel right now like a person who hasn't been sick a day in his life," Davis was quoted in *The Los Angeles Times* on December 18, 1963, after appearing at a press conference a month and a half after his kidney transplant.[11] "I had no choice. The doctors told me I couldn't live with what I got. A monkey's kidney don't bother me in any way. All I wanted to do was survive." Reemtsma was also quoted, saying, "perhaps most significant is that the transplanted chimpanzee's kidneys not only functioned when first put in, but . . . went through a phase of rejection and then continued to function." He also "emphasized that the operation was undertaken with the patient's consent only after a careful explanation that the chances for success were unpredictable."

On December 18th, Davis was discharged home. Jefferson Davis, father of four, had been an inpatient for six and a half months, much of it on dialysis. He received a chimpanzee transplant, in an era when human transplants were rare. He was successfully treated through two potential rejection crises before it was known that rejection could be treated even in human kidneys. And he was going home.

The celebratory feelings faded only two days later, when he was readmitted with high fevers. His kidney function was normal, but he looked sick. Pneumonia was diagnosed by clinical exam and x-ray. Attempts were made to reduce his immunosuppression, but he rapidly developed shock due to sepsis (infection that became systemic). On January 7th, Jefferson Davis died of pneumonia, eighteen days after his readmission and sixty-three days after his transplant. An autopsy confirmed his pneumonia. Other than some acute injury to the kidneys from his lung infection, his transplanted chimpanzee kidneys looked healthy. There were no signs of rejection on pathologic exam. Although this was a tragic outcome, it was no worse than those being achieved with human organs. The knowledge that rejection was prevented provided hope to the team about the potential for xenotransplantation. Reemtsma was devastated, but he felt justified to continue his efforts, as nothing about the Davis case seemed insurmountable. He still believed xeno could offer hope to his patients who had no other options.

His next patient was a twelve-year-old boy who had undergone multiple operations to fix a chronic blockage where his kidneys drained into his bladder. When Reemtsma performed the transplant on this boy, using the same technique as he did on Davis, he discovered how abnormal the boy's bladder really was. The boy developed a urine leak and, despite the best efforts by the team, died seven weeks later from infection, with beautifully functioning kidneys. This was a crushing loss for everyone involved.

On January 13, 1964, just six days after Jefferson Davis's death, Reemtsma performed his third chimpanzee xenotransplant into a young woman he had been taking care of for over two months. Twenty-three-year-old Edith Parker was a schoolteacher from Napoleonville, Louisiana. She was admitted in November 1963 with chronic kidney disease and was placed on emergent dialysis. She remained in the hospital until a blood group–and size-matched chimpanzee became available. Her transplant worked immediately and made seven liters of urine in the first twenty-four hours. Her kidney function and blood pressure normalized within the first couple of days. She suffered a suspected rejection episode twenty-three days after transplant, which was reversed with irradiation and increased immunosuppression. She was ultimately released from the hospital and even returned to teaching in

September 1964. Now Reemtsma had two xeno recipients that made it home. Although this seemed to be a massive success, he remained cautious when talking to patients and the press.

Reemtsma's next three xenotransplant patients proved to be extremely challenging. He performed four sets of chimpanzee transplants into three patients (one had to be retransplanted two days after the first transplant, as the grafts never worked). All of the patients died from a combination of rejection and infection in under a month, with Reemtsma and his entire team spending almost the entirety of that time at their bedsides. The last patient was a sixteen-year-old girl, and her death was particularly difficult for the team to manage emotionally. They were exhausted.

There was much to be excited about from this trial, but in the end, six of the seven patients that received primate transplants were dead. Then there was Edith Parker, the third patient to receive the chimpanzee xenotransplant, who was back to her normal routine at home. It was this patient's remarkable success that energized the entire team, keeping them going when things seemed so dark. Parker was seen in the clinic weekly, which hardly seemed necessary given how well she looked. Unfortunately, that wasn't to last. More than nine months after her transplant, Edith Parker died. On the day before her death, she was admitted for a twenty-four-hour illness of undetermined etiology, and died while in the hospital. Her kidneys were functioning well until the end. At autopsy, there was no evidence of rejection. Sadly, Reemtsma was in New York at the time of her death. He had just presented her case at a conference sponsored by the National Kidney Disease Foundation. He was personally devastated.

Reemtsma was considering another series of chimpanzee transplants. But this wasn't to be. By 1965, options were improving for transplant patients. Outcomes with living and deceased donor kidneys were improving. Long-term dialysis was becoming a reality. Despite Reemtsma's belief that chimpanzees could be a viable option for human transplant, he made clear that it was experimental, and made sure his patients understood that he couldn't predict what the outcomes might be. He always ensured the patients had no access to living donors and no imminent offers for deceased donors—in other words, that this experimental treatment was their best, and probably only, option. Once the availability of deceased donors increased, and the potential for chronic dialysis became a reality, he moved his work on xeno into the lab rather than the clinic. He could no longer justify such an experimental procedure when his patients increasingly had other options. As he said years later, "I picked a window in history when it was ethically acceptable to do this. No one had any success in cadaveric grafts, and nobody had dialysis. The patients, if they didn't have a brother or sister to donate a kidney, had nothing."[12] Even if Reemtsma couldn't provide them much of a chance of a long-term survival, at least he could offer them hope.

Reemtsma was not secretive about the transplants he was performing, and the public reaction to the cases was extremely positive. Cases were followed by press releases and were covered extensively in the lay press nationwide, from small, local journals to *The New York Times* and *Newsweek*. Reemtsma would always get his first update on how his patients were doing on the drive into the hospital, as the cases and status of the patients would be discussed on the morning radio shows. His archival collection is filled with letters from elementary to high school students from across the United States and the world, asking about the transplants and how the patients were doing. Each archived letter was accompanied by a copy of a response from his office promising more information as it became available.

Reemtsma never faced any major protests, threats, or negativity from the public regarding his use of primates or his "experimental" transplants on humans while at Tulane. He did, however, face criticism from other physicians and ethicists at meetings and in the press, accusing him of taking too much risk with his patients and not focusing enough on the outcomes. Reemtsma always highlighted the importance of extensive discussions with the patient and their family about their wishes, discussions that he always documented carefully. He would state publicly that "no individual is ever forced to take a transplant. Every patient has a right to die, and some choose to do so."[13]

Reemtsma never attempted any more clinical solid organ xenotransplants after this first series, but his influence on the field of surgery, transplant, organ replacement, and xenotransplantation was only just beginning. In 1966, he became the chair of surgery at the University of Utah. In 1971,

Reemtsma left Utah to become the chair of surgery at the Columbia University College of Physicians and Surgeons in New York, where he had gone to medical school. He remained chair there until 1994. Reemtsma was seen by everyone who worked with him as a visionary and an indefatigable optimist with a remarkable sense of humor. He surrounded himself with great people and empowered them to innovate with his support. They felt comfortable taking risks and pushing limits because Reemtsma was always there to protect them and shut down the naysayers. Did he develop this attitude during his free rein riding horseback with his Navajo friends in Fort Defiance? Or did it come from his experience in Korea as a fresh young trainee flouting the rules and risking court martial to do what he knew was right? Reemtsma never gave an answer to that.

One thing that is clear about the man, however, is that he was absolutely beloved by everyone who trained with him, worked with him, was taken care of by him, or knew him. Every one of his mentees with whom I spoke stated that he was the single most important person in their lives, beyond their spouses (and a few didn't mention their spouses). Any surgeon who met Reemtsma wanted to work with him—and be like him. A famous Reemtsma quote was "Surround yourself with good people, get out of their way, and borrow their slides on occasion." Reemtsma was larger than life, always wearing his cowboy hat and boots from his days on the reservation. At the end of every transplant, Reemtsma would poke his trainee in the ribs and deliver his favorite quote, "Another Goddamn Miracle." Because that's what transplant is—a miracle.

* * * * *

Reemtsma's efforts in New Orleans did not go unnoticed in the small transplant community, and he was happy to share his results with anyone who was interested. His two most illustrious visitors were James Hardy from Mississippi and Tom Starzl from Denver. Reemtsma jokingly "described the two famous visiting surgeons taking copious notes while in New Orleans, rushing to their return trains, and getting off near the zoos in their respective cities to reserve and recruit any available chimpanzees or baboons."[14] Hardy described his impressions years later. "They had two patients in the hospital at that time, one of whom was a young female schoolteacher who had had a chimpanzee kidney transplant some seven months previously. She was doing surprisingly well, and there was a man there who was also doing pretty well. So I decided that, if they can do this at Tulane, *we* could give it a try. After all, we had nothing else to offer. There was no chronic dialysis then. We bought four large chimpanzees, and had them available for kidney transplants."[15] James Hardy gets only a footnote in historical discussions of the evolution of transplant, even though he performed the first recorded lung transplant in a human in April of 1963 (which failed after eighteen days), and then half a year later the first heart transplant ever placed in a human on the morning of January 24, 1964. It was a chimpanzee heart, placed in the chest of a dying man who was too sick and too big for that heart to have a chance. The heart beat well initially, but it was too weak to sustain life, and after ninety minutes, the man died on the table.

Starzl is best known for his work in liver transplantation, a field he single-handedly made a reality through massive effort and persistence. But he also saw potential in Reemtsma's transplants and became a devotee to xenotransplantation. In 1964, he performed six baboon-to-human kidney transplants into recipients that had no potential living donors, were on dialysis, and couldn't find deceased donors. The recipients lived nineteen to ninety-eights days but ultimately succumbed to some combination of rejection and infection.

In the pathologic analysis, Starzl and his team was able to compare the pathology from Reemtsma's series of chimpanzees to his own experience with baboons, and there was a dramatic difference. The chimpanzee kidneys showed minimal signs of rejection, no worse than what would normally be seen in human-to-human transplants, while the baboon kidneys showed severe damage from rejection.[16] "The death of six patients was a devastating loss. We never tried again."[17]

He never tried again with kidney transplants. But livers were different. In July of 1966 Starzl implanted a chimpanzee liver into a twenty-eight-month-old child with a failing liver. The chimpanzee liver worked right away but the child died of infection after nine days. This was no different than what was seen with human liver transplantation at that time. The first successful liver transplant (lasting more than a year) wouldn't occur until 1967, performed by Starzl himself.[18]

Outcomes remained horrific for another decade and a half. He attempted two more chimpanzee liver transplants, one in 1969 and one in 1973. Both patients died shortly after surgery, but Starzl blamed himself rather than the fact that the donors were chimpanzees. He remained convinced that chimpanzee-to-human transplantation had potential, but felt it shouldn't be attempted again until better immunosuppression was available.[19] The rest of the transplant community followed his lead. Xenotransplantation would need to wait until the ability to suppress the immune response was improved.

2 BABY FAE AND THE END OF THE PRIMATE ERA (1984–1988)

If you mention the name Baby Fae to most people in their sixties or older, they will remember the name, although perhaps not the details or why it was important. It was forty years ago that this innocent, courageous baby underwent the most famous xenotransplantation ever performed. The world was captivated by her story. But the controversy surrounding the transplant, the surgeon, her parents, and the choice of donor rocked the world of xeno. Some of the accusations that flew in the aftermath were grounded in falsehoods and disinformation. This case forever changed the course of xenotransplantation, marking the end of the use of primates as a source of organs for humans. It remains the most widely known attempt at saving someone's life with the use of an animal organ.

Barstow, California, October 14, 1984

When Teresa Beauclair first noticed vaginal bleeding, she knew it was time to go to the hospital.[1] She was already thirty-eight weeks pregnant, certainly enough time to have a healthy baby. But she was still worried. The pregnancy had been straightforward, just like her last one with her son Beau, now a healthy toddler. Her relationship with her boyfriend, Howard, had been more complicated. The two had split up just a few weeks before. So when Teresa rushed to the hospital, she was alone.

Within three hours of arriving at the small local hospital, the baby was born. It was a girl, and she was uncommonly beautiful. Teresa picked out the name Stephanie, after her favorite actor Stephanie Powers. Ironically, Powers was starring in the television series *Hart to Hart* at the time. Teresa only held her new daughter for a minute before they whisked her out of the delivery room. Something wasn't right. They didn't know what it was, but they knew she needed to be at a bigger hospital. Baby Stephanie was driven the seventy-six miles, alone, to the medical center in Loma Linda, California.

As soon as Teresa was discharged from the hospital, she rushed to join her baby. It was there that Teresa was told that her daughter had hypoplastic left heart syndrome, meaning the left side of her heart was underdeveloped and wouldn't be strong enough to pump oxygenated blood to her vital organs. She was going to die.

Teresa had three options. She could let her baby die in the hospital at Loma Linda, she could transfer her back to the community hospital in Barstow to die, or she could take her home to die. Teresa was shell shocked. She knew she didn't want her baby to die in the hospital, but she also didn't want her to die in her home, with her son Beau there. So she took Stephanie, and checked into a motel in Barstow. Her mom came into town to take care of Beau, and in that motel, alone with this perfect and yet fatally flawed baby, she fell in love. She would do everything in her power to keep her baby alive as long as possible.

After a couple of days, Teresa noticed that Stephanie's eyes were turning yellow, and she called the neonatologist back at Loma Linda to let him know. The neonatologist had a surprising suggestion. A pediatric cardiac surgeon by the name of Dr. Leonard Bailey had returned to town and might have something experimental to offer. If Teresa was interested, he would set up a consultation. She was interested, and the two set up a meeting in a conference room at Loma Linda. Teresa did reach out to Stephanie's father to see if he could come, but he wasn't available. He asked Teresa to record it, so she brought a tape recorder and recorded the seven-hour consultation in its entirety. Seven hours. It was during that time that Dr. Bailey shared with Teresa his efforts to devise a treatment plan for babies like Stephanie.

* * * * *

Bailey first became intrigued with the idea of transplantation when he was a medical student at Loma Linda. He visited Stanford in the late 1960s, just as cardiac transplantation was in its infancy. He was able to go to Norm Shumway's lab, where he saw the master himself perform experimental heart transplants in dogs. Shumway would perform the first "successful" heart transplant in the United States, on January 6, 1968. The recipient, a fifty-four-year-old man, would live for fourteen days. Heart transplant outcomes were dismal in those early years, and it would be a decade and a half before heart transplantation would become a reliable treatment option for patients with end-stage cardiac disease (a recurring comment for the early experience with transplant).

Bailey found himself simultaneously fascinated with heart transplantation and pediatric surgery. As he conducted his training in surgery at Toronto's Hospital for Sick Children, he had the opportunity to take care of many babies and children that died from congenital heart disease. As he remarked about those children in the 1970s, ". . . at that time, babies born with certain kinds of exotic heart disease weren't even treated—they were set aside to die. And they uniformly did that."[2] Bailey saw the reconstructive operations that were being attempted on these infants as palliative. He had little interest in that. He knew there had to be a better way.

Specifically, he believed that better way was replacement of the entire heart. But after the initial excitement that cardiac transplant had inspired in the late 1960s, leading to hundreds of heart transplant performed across the country (all adults), the sad reality was setting in. Almost all of these patients were dying of rejection. Bailey was aware, from experience in the lab in Toronto, that newborns had "primitive" immune systems compared to adults. In his own words, the newborn immune system ". . . has very little of the aggressiveness of the older child or an adult. It has no experience, which helps. And much of the suppressor type behavior is still intact in the newborn. So the possibility that a newborn could receive a graft and actually grow up without any immune suppression was curious enough."

When Bailey returned to Loma Linda University Medical Center as a faculty member in 1976, he revitalized the cardiac research lab. He obtained funding from the department at the medical school and hired a team of technicians to help with the experiments and the animal care. He focused on newborn goats as his recipients, and used goats and lambs to serve as donors.[3] He had a nearby farm facility where the animals were housed.

The first set of experiments tested the hypothesis that infants had such an immature immune system that they could accept transplants without any immunosuppression. Bailey and his team would take a baby goat that was just a few days old and perform an orthotopic heart transplant. He would remove the heart of the newborn (after he put the goat on a cardiac bypass machine), and sew a heart from a different unrelated goat of the same age into the same spot where the old heart sat—and let it recover. No immunosuppression was administered. It was known from both animal models and experience in humans that adult recipients of non-identical hearts would reject the organs within a week. But in Bailey's experiments in the newborns, within a week they would be back at the farm jumping around with the other goats. The animals thrived at first, but ultimately would suffer terminal rejection. The average survival in this series was fifty-three days with one living six months, which was remarkable given that no immunosuppression was used.

Bailey then transplanted lamb hearts into baby goats without immunosuppression and observed an average survival of six days. The hearts were acutely rejected, showing that neonatal goat immune systems had the ability to mount an aggressive immune response and reject xenotransplants. Bailey tried both sets of experiments (goat-to-goat and lamb-to-goat) with the immunosuppression available at the time (azathioprine and prednisone), but didn't see dramatic improvement in outcomes.

In the early 1980s, word began to travel through the transplant community about a new and extremely powerful pharmaceutical agent that had been isolated from soil samples. Cyclosporine, so named because of the molecule's cyclic structure, was a natural product of fungi that was identified when employees of the pharmaceutical company Sandoz (now Novartis) returned from a Norwegian vacation with the soil samples in tow. This may sound like an odd souvenir from a family vacation, but Sandoz had a program in place encouraging employees to collect such samples to be analyzed as they searched for antibiotic properties of fungal metabolites. Cyclosporine had a remarkable ability to suppress the function of T cells, a primary cell of the immune system. It was first used in transplantation by Roy Calne in the

United Kingdom, followed by Starzl in Denver. Cyclosporine, used at the right dose and combined with steroids, had the ability to minimize rejection episodes while having a tolerable side-effect profile. In 1983, the drug would receive FDA approval for use in transplantation, and would transform the field overnight, essentially doubling patient survival to 90 percent at one year. More than anything, this wonder drug was the reason transplantation would go from an experimental field to a reliable treatment option for patients with organ failure.

A few years before its approval, as Calne and Shumway were trialing cyclosporine in humans, Bailey reached out to John Borel, the scientist at Sandoz leading the efforts with the drug. Bailey asked Borel if he could get a supply for his pediatric experiments, and Borel agreed. Bailey performed a series of goat-to-goat orthotopic heart transplants in neonates, with daily cyclosporine administration. They lived indefinitely, just on the single immunosuppressive drug. He used goats from the same herd, and then outbred goats, representing a different subspecies (of which there are many). "That took our breath away—the fact that we could transplant a baby at birth and have that baby grow up with nothing more than receiving injections of this oily substance. The baby goats would go down to the farm, grow up, become big herd animals, and actually grow old. And if they didn't get in trouble, they would die just of old age."[4]

The results convinced Bailey that cardiac transplantation in the newborn would become a reality. He was building up a referral base of children with hypoplastic left heart syndrome and other congenital defects that led to certain death. He was absolutely convinced that the only way to save these babies would be heart transplantation, and now he knew it could be done. But he had no access to donors. There was no national system to identify donors in the early 1980s, and his own efforts had been fruitless. Whenever he consulted on a baby with the diagnosis of hypoplastic left heart, he knew he had just a few days to find a donor, which proved to be impossible. They would all just die. Bailey turned his attention in the lab to xenotransplantation. He performed a series of lamb hearts into goats using cyclosporine. In his first reported series, fourteen newborn goats received orthotopic lamb hearts and were treated with cyclosporine, steroids, and azathioprine, the strongest immunosuppressive regimen available. Ten of the goats lived through the operation. Survival of those ten recipients averaged seventy-two days, with one animal surviving 165 days. Bailey also tried a series of piglet hearts to goats and achieved a more modest thirty-one-day survival. Bailey concluded that closer-matched xenotransplant pairs had the potential to survive longer after transplant.

Bailey didn't have access to any chimps, gorillas, or other apes, as these animals, unlike baboons, were either protected or rare. This made them very costly—far too expensive for Bailey to consider using. He was convinced that a cross-species transplant into a human baby could work. More than anything, Bailey wanted to transplant human hearts into these babies, but despite his efforts, he had no human donors. Bailey and his team began to investigate the biology of a group of olive baboons, the most common baboon available to researchers in the United States. He screened the baboons for infectious diseases, excluding those that carried any known viruses that could infect human recipients. He then performed numerous immunologic assays using human blood, characterizing potential immune responses that could lead to rejection after transplantation. He became more convinced that the infant immune system would have a mild response to a baboon organ, a response he could temper with available immunosuppression.

The final thing Bailey examined was blood type. He knew that baboons rarely have blood type O, the universal donor. Bailey did test all of the baboons he had available for their blood type, and the majority had blood type AB, the most common type found in baboons. Humans have antibodies in their blood for the blood-type groups they don't carry, so patients with O blood type will have antibodies against group A and B antigens. The importance of blood-type compatibility was still somewhat unclear in the early 1980s, and there were examples of blood-type-incompatible organ transplants that had succeeded. Almost nothing was known about transplanting infants in this era. It was well recognized that infants have very little antibody present in their serum, and they do not produce ABO antibodies until three to six months of age. In addition, the infant blood group is expressed at very low levels in newborns, which is protective as blood group antibodies can cross the placenta during pregnancy. Given all of this, and the challenge of finding blood-type-O baboons, Bailey thought he might consider using a baboon heart in a baby human across a blood-type incompatible barrier, as long as the other immunologic tests were promising.

These data led Bailey to approach the Loma Linda University Institutional Review Board (IRB) (a relatively new entity to approve potentially risky novel treatments) to apply for approval to perform baboon-to-human neonatal heart transplants. The process took fourteen months, and included opinions from external reviewers from the various fields related to transplantation and immunology. Multiple resubmissions with extensive revisions were required, but ultimately his protocol was approved. He would be cleared to perform five cross-species heart transplants into infants. Bailey was finally ready to move into humans.

* * * * *

Bailey had just returned to Loma Linda after a brief trip when he was stopped in the hall by a cardiologist he knew well. "'You know, Bailey, how's that protocol coming? I happen to have a baby in the nursery now with this problem. Are you interested?' I said, 'Well, let me do some checking.' I got back to him and said, 'Yes, I think we are.'"[5]

Shortly after the encounter, Bailey found himself in a consultation room with Teresa Beauclair and her tape recorder. For the next seven hours, Bailey told Teresa about all of his research making sure she understood it was all in non-human animals. He explained that it was experimental, had never been done in humans, and he really couldn't say if her baby would survive and for how long. He was confident he could get her through the operation, and it was his personal belief that her baby could survive well beyond that. He was not proposing it as a bridge to a human transplant, but as her destination therapy. He believed Stephanie could live many years with a baboon heart.

He told Teresa about the reconstructive operations that existed at the time, which he described as palliative. He did not offer them as an option, as he thought they didn't work and Stephanie was too old to qualify even if he did perform them.

Teresa's first reaction was relatable. "I wondered if the doctor was a mad scientist."[6] At the end of the conference, Teresa did agree to let Bailey begin testing her baby's blood against the twelve baboons that he had available for a potential transplant. According to the policy approved by the IRB, a second consent to conduct these tests had to be completed twenty-four hours later. Teresa gave her consent a second time.

Blood was drawn from baby Stephanie, and the immunologic testing began. The results were reviewed by one of Bailey's collaborators, Dr. Sandra Nehlsen-Cannarella, an external consultant who had weighed in when the IRB was conducting its review. Of the twelve baboons, Stephanie's blood clearly showed that one in particular, a nine-month-old female named Goobers, was the most compatible. As they conducted the workup, Stephanie was becoming visibly sicker, with an awful blue hue and an inability to eat. They set the surgery for October 26, 1984, a Friday, just one day after the final immunologic testing was complete. When Bailey discussed the final details of the operation with Teresa, he explained that there likely would be significant interest from the press. They both thought it might be safest to use a pseudonym for Stephanie. They would use her middle name, Fae. She would be referred to as Baby Fae.

As the morning of the transplant approached, Bailey wasn't nervous at all. He had done so many newborn transplants in the lab, along with countless complex heart surgeries on adults and children. He was a confident, supremely talented heart surgeon.

Bailey was in the animal lab by six o'clock the next morning, where he met with his team to make sure they had all the details in place. He was rested, calm, confident, ready to go. Just another day of heart surgery.

Bailey and his team started with Goobers, opening her chest and exposing her perfectly healthy nine-month-old beating heart. He placed his clamps and removed the heart like he had done so many times before in the lab. He brought the heart up to the main OR, where Baby Fae was already asleep, prepped and draped on the table. He made his incision, opened her sternum, and got to work. As was the case for all the pioneering surgeons who came before Bailey, and those who would come after, no amount of preparation would allow him to anticipate the creativity that would be required to overcome the anomalous physiology that he would encounter. "We'd done it so many times, although we'd never really worked with hypoplastic left heart syndrome. It cast a slightly different nuance on the surgery, because the whole aortic arch had to be reconstructed as part of the process. We had dreamt of how it might go, but we'd never actually done it in exactly this way in a baby."[7]

Bailey had no problem improvising. "We were blessed. It just turned out beautifully. Her response to the surgery was just perfect." The heart was a perfect size, made to order. Everything matched up beautifully, and Bailey sewed it in expertly. Baby Fae's new heart began beating spontaneously on rewarming. No electric shock was required. The heart seemed not to care that it would now function in a different species. The heart quickly increased its contractions to 130 beats per minute, normal for a baby. The crowd that was present in the OR erupted in excitement. "There was absolute awe," remarked Nehlsen-Cannarella years later.[8] "I don't think there was a dry eye in the room." To everyone present, it truly seemed to be a miracle. Baby Fae was returned to the ICU to begin her recovery in fantastic shape.

Bailey and his team knew there would be coverage in the press. He knew that there would be some naysayers, people second-guessing his choices, probably some animal rights activists protesting. But the actual reaction was so far beyond his wildest dreams, including his nightmares. "I didn't think that Baby Fae's transplant would set off so many alarms. I thought there might be some regional interest, but the story became world news. That part of it was a little surprising. And it was a bit of a distraction—it did affect her care. We felt like we were operating in a glass bowl."[9]

The coverage in the press was immense. It was front page in every newspaper, and the lead story on every television program across the country. The nation was gripped with excitement over this miracle, thirsting for constant updates on Baby Fae's condition. The reaction wasn't all positive. Animal rights activists converged in Loma Linda to protest the "ghoulish tinkering with human and animal life." The protesters were shown on television carrying signs that read, "Animal Research Is Scientific Fraud," "Animal Experiments Never Cured Anything," "Animal Researchers Are Quacks." The attacks on Bailey were personal, accusing him of choosing to sacrifice Goober for his own career advancement. Death threats poured in threatening Bailey and his family. He was assigned a police detail, and his family had to have round-the-clock protection. "My family suffered immensely," he said. "We had to have police live in our home, for instance. Our personal mail was opened by the police department for over a year. I wasn't allowed to appear in public without a bullet-proof vest under my clothing because of the array of threats that came through in those days."[10]

Bailey wasn't immune to the ethical challenges of sacrificing a baboon to save a human. But he was resolute in his belief that he would do anything to save his patients. "Some say that the animal's life is just as valuable as the human baby's life and that we have no business taking the animal's life. I'm sensitive to that point of view, I have some misgivings about it myself. But as I look at the planet earth and the various species that are scattered about, there is a certain survival of the fittest that goes on in nature, the lion eats the zebra and so forth, and it seems to me, as a human being, that my obligation is to my own species first. If there is a way to support the life of a member of my own species, even though it requires the sensitive and caring taking of a subhuman primate life, I think I'm obligated to pursue that course of action."[11]

It wasn't just animal rights activists who protested Bailey. The medical bioethics community voiced major reservations for what Bailey had done. They questioned whether Bailey had practiced informed consent with the parents, and specifically on what was written on consent forms that Teresa signed before surgery. They questioned whether Bailey had offered Teresa reconstructive procedures. They questioned whether Bailey had attempted to obtain a human heart. He did not offer the baboon transplant as a bridge to human transplantation. He didn't see the xenotransplant as a temporary measure, a palliative option. He saw it as a cure. He would have loved to give Baby Fae a human heart instead of a baboon, but did not believe it was realistic to find an appropriately sized donor in the limited time the infant could wait. All of his previous attempts at this had been failures. In the early 1980s, cardiac transplantation was a very limited business, and other than one single failed attempt in 1968, no baby had ever undergone a heart transplant.

Many of Bailey's colleagues were vocally critical as well. "One surgeon observed that the child's chances of survival would have been equally served if Bailey had dispensed with the baboon—and sewn in an alarm clock."[12] A number of prominent transplant surgeons predicted imminent failure and death. They criticized Bailey's limited numbers of publications in scientific journals regarding his xeno data. Many in the field assumed he had jumped in and performed the xenotransplant with no preparation whatsoever.

The saddest, most despicable part of the press reaction to the story is how it handled Teresa. The hospital had done everything it could to keep secret the identity of "Fae's" parents, but ultimately the press tracked Teresa down. News outlets didn't initially publish Teresa Beauclair's name, but they focused on her character, disparaging her and her husband whenever they could. "NBC has learned the identity of the child's parents. We will respect their wishes and not name them. However, certain aspects of their past might be relevant to some of the medical controversies in this case. According to relatives and court records, the couple were never married. They had separated by the time the infant was born. Both had been in trouble with the law in the state they came from, the father for disorderly conduct, the mother for passing bad checks. They had little money when the child was born." In multiple reports, the press referred to Teresa as ignorant, illiterate, ill informed, drug addicted. This was an awful time for Teresa, who just wanted to be left alone and be with her baby.

Despite all of the criticism and character assassination, the one person that seemed to be unbothered and thriving was Baby Fae. For two weeks, she did beautifully. The breathing tube was removed, and she was photographed happily enjoying a bottle and smiling for the press. "Nine days after the operation, with Baby Fae seemingly doing fine, Bailey enthusiastically predicted that Fae might celebrate her 20th birthday. He predicted that Goober's heart would grow as Fae grew." "On November 4th [postoperative day 9] she was offered full-strength formula for the first time since the operation. The next day they reported that she was eating normally, grasping at objects and wailing with a lusty cry."[13]

It wouldn't last. On postoperative day sixteen, she started to show signs of rejection, and the cyclosporine was increased. On day seventeen, she had to be placed back on the ventilator and fed through an IV. She continued to worsen and finally died on postoperative day twenty-one.[14] Bailey held a press conference. "Today we grieve the loss of this precious life . . . which could have been an absolute loss to her loved ones . . . her unique place in our memories will derive from what she and her parents have done to give rise to a ray of hope for the babies to come."[15] Years later, Teresa Beauclair told an interviewer, "The night that Stephanie died I asked Dr. Bailey to not let this experience be wasted, and to keep going forward with it."[16]

It wasn't initially clear why Baby Fae died. Analysis of the heart at autopsy showed minimal evidence of T-cell rejection, the standard type of rejection typically seen in human-to-human transplantation. There was some evidence of swelling and injury to the heart, likely secondary to antibody, which was presumed to be directed at the mismatch in blood type despite Fae being an infant.

Bailey was both surprised and crushed when Baby Fae died. He really believed she would live, especially when he saw how beautifully the donor heart performed in the OR. He spent almost every second of those three weeks at Fae's bedside, or with Teresa. Even years later, he remained confused about why the heart ultimately failed. In a recent analysis of the case, it was noted that early after transplant, Baby Fae received an overdose of cyclosporine, and her blood had to be cleansed of the drug with pheresis, a system that filters blood by running it through a machine. As her blood was replaced, she received an infusion that includes human serum, and it has been suggested that perhaps this serum contained antibodies that rejected the baboon graft. It's a plausible theory, but in the end remains just that. As Bailey said in an interview more than twenty years later, "To this day, it's a bit of a mystery what went on. Anyhow, she died, and that was heartbreaking. We invested a lot of time, energy, and effort. We had gotten to know her family . . . The hate mail and threats poured in for a long time, so much so that the Redlands police wanted us to let them open our mail and things like that . . . We had two little children, Connor and Brooks, who were quite impressed when the police came up to the house and gave us all lessons about how to take care of ourselves."[17]

Initially, Bailey had plans to do four more xenotransplants from baboons, but he hesitated. He had put his family through so much, and himself suffered so much criticism from colleagues around the world. Although he had no regrets when it came to Baby Fae and Teresa, he did recognize that portions of the public and medical community may not have been ready for what he did. "I am not sure that I know where I stand on this. I take a lead from my children. Neither they nor I like the idea of taking the lives of healthy primates and the only way we can justify it is the notion that we can save a member of our own species . . . It gives you pause for reflection. You have to continually check what you are doing against public opinion, whether or not it is justifiable, whether it is right."[18]

At the same time, he believed that bold steps had to be taken to push a field forward, or perhaps just to save the patient he had in front of him. He was willing to do what he believed in, and to pay whatever price he had to if he felt he was in the right. "There are very few free-wheeling immunologists, and immunology, while fascinating, is an imperfect science. It takes a bold surgeon to put immunology to the test. The immunologists want to get all their ducks in a row before they act, and the surgeon, who must deal with dying babies, does not have that luxury. You can't always armchair this debate. There are some very practical considerations that need to be put to the test. The surgeon must act."[19]

In the end, the success of new opportunities—directly related to Baby Fae—prevented Bailey from doing another baboon-to-human transplant. He had another baby in the hospital, Eddie, who also had a failing heart from hypoplastic left heart syndrome. Eddie was clearly going to die. But then Bailey got a call from an obstetrician in the Bay Area. "I know what you did for Baby Fae. Are you still doing transplants, because I have a baby here with birth asphyxia, and the parents want the baby's organs donated. Nobody else wants baby organs except you." Bailey responded, "Well, I think we do want that heart."[20]

Eddie's parents wanted to move forward, having lost another child one year prior with a similar heart condition. Shortly thereafter, Bailey conducted the world's first successful neonatal heart transplant. They gave Eddie a temporary moniker, Baby Moses, knowing the press would quickly return to Loma Linda to see what Bailey was up to. "When we did the first allograft transplant a year later with Baby Moses, wouldn't you know there were several busloads of people who came out to picket the house. The Redlands police, stars that they are, only permitted these people to demonstrate in front of our neighbors' house."[21] The press arrived in force, covering the story with the same vigor as before, initially reporting that the donor was another baboon. Public interest remained focused even after it was discovered that the donor was a human baby, because Baby Moses, like Fae, kept getting better and better.

Baby Moses, now known to be Eddie Anguiano, is still alive today! He is the longest-living recipient of an infant heart transplant in the world.

Bailey credits the heroism of Fae and her family for allowing Eddie to survive, and for the development of a system to allocate infant and baby hearts for transplant. Bailey built one of the largest pediatric heart transplant programs in the world, saving the lives of hundreds of babies and children over his long and successful career. In the final tally, Bailey transplanted hearts into 376 infants over his forty-two-year career at Loma Linda, with excellent outcomes. He continued to perform xenotransplants in the laboratory, but never again in humans. After seeing the firestorm of criticism that Bailey faced, virtually everyone in the xeno world retreated to the laboratory as well.

* * * * *

As the twenty-fifth anniversary of Reemtsma's chimp-to-human kidney transplants approached, transplant surgeon Mark Hardy had an idea. Having been recruited by then-chairman of surgery Reemtsma to Columbia-Presbyterian Hospital in New York City in the 1970s, where he had founded the abdominal transplant program, Hardy decided to organize an international conference to celebrate the twenty-fifth anniversary of Reemtsma's first successful xenotransplant in man. His vision was to have a two-day conference in a secluded location to allow uninhibited discussion of the science, the data, the successes, and the failures. He also wanted to address the ethical and social aspects of the field. He thought hard about who to include at this meeting, which would also host Starzl, Roy Calne, and Reemtsma himself.

As Hardy considered the events surrounding Baby Fae, including the vitriol that Bailey and his team experienced, one name came to his mind. He pulled out his stationary and penned a letter. It started simply "Dear Ms.

Goodall." He addressed the letter to Jane Goodall's foundation. It might seem strange that Hardy invited her to this meeting celebrating xenotransplantation, as she obviously was not going to be sympathetic to the idea of breeding primates, chimpanzees in particular, to transplant organs into human recipients. "I thought she was a critical part of the story." Goodall agreed. She accepted the invitation to the conference.

The meeting was held on November 11–13, 1988, at Arden House, Harriman, New York. The house was owned by a railroad magnate Edward Henry Harriman at the turn of the twentieth century, and now serves as a conference center. It sits atop a mountain outside the town of Harriman, New York, about forty miles northwest of Manhattan. The meeting commenced with consecutive talks from Sir Roy Calne, Keith Reemtsma, and Tom Starzl. They each recounted their own experiences with xenotransplantation beginning in the early 1960s. Of the three, Calne was the most incredulous about the future of xenotransplantation as a clinical reality. Starzl was slightly more optimistic but also realistic about the challenges that still existed. Reemtsma was the most optimistic of the holy trinity of speakers.

After this first session, what followed was two days' worth of talks from the experts, the people doing the basic research on experimental models, organ physiology of different animals, immunology and genetics, manipulation of organs, and then finally a session on the social, ethical, legal, and political issues facing the field. It was in this session that Jane Goodall gave her talk, titled "Ethical concerns in the use of animals as donors."

Goodall jumped right into the fray, discussing her concerns about using animals for research.[22] "The more we learn of the true nature of non-human animals, especially of those with complex brains and correspondingly complex social behavior, the more does this raise ethical concerns regarding their use in the service of man—whether this be for entertainment, as 'pets,' in research laboratories or any of the other uses to which we subject them." She next addressed accusations against her that she believed misrepresented her opinions about the importance of animal research. "I have been described as a 'rabid anti-vivisectionist.' My counter to that is that my own mother is alive today because her clogged aortic valve was removed and replaced by that of a pig. The valve in question . . . came, we were told, from a commercially slaughtered hog. In other words, the pig would have died anyway. This, however, does not eliminate my ethical concern as regards that pig in particular or pigs in general. The manner in which pigs are maintained commercially today, in the intensive farming units, is morally unacceptable to me. I hope, at some point, to be able to influence public opinion on that regard. And I want to fight for more humane treatment of laboratory pigs." Goodall stated that she understood if all animal research were abruptly stopped, that would cause confusion and chaos in the world of science and medicine, and would ultimately increase human suffering. But she hoped that the numbers of animals needed for research could be greatly reduced.

Goodall then moved on to describe her relationship with the chimpanzees, discussing her experience over the past twenty-nine years observing one particular group of them in the Gombe National Park in Tanzania. She talked about them as if they were part of her own family, knowing their names, personalities, and character flaws. She described their relationships, their intellect, their ability to love, be sad, fight, be scared. She talked about their use of tools and even sign language. She recalled their happiness when a newborn chimp was welcomed to the family, and their sadness when a family member died (not just sadness, but even clinical depression). She told stories of Flo, that "tolerant, affectionate, protective and playful mother." Of neurotic Flint, a spoiled brat who insisted even at the age of six that his mother carry him, and who died of grief when she died. Of twelve-year-old Spindle, who adopted the orphaned Mel, sharing food and nest. Of Mike, who became the alpha male despite his small size, by means of his brain: He taught himself to menace the other males by rushing at them kicking three empty kerosene cans all at once, which made such a gaudy racket that he never had to fight. Goodall closed with the tale of Old Man, a chimpanzee in Florida who saved his keeper's life, protecting the man from other chimpanzees. "We humans might care to reciprocate, she suggested."

The audience was stunned. It was much easier to listen to talks about graft survival, surgical technique, immunosuppression, treatment of rejection. This was something different altogether, coming after two days of presentations about the future of this exciting field. After the meeting, there was consensus that chimpanzees were not going to serve as donors for human transplantation, or recipients in animal models. There was still some disagreement on baboons and other monkeys. At the very least, they would need to serve as recipients in laboratory studies as a model for the human recipient. Starzl ended his own talk with a story that was particularly relevant:

"About 5 years ago, I approached the NIH a month or 6 weeks before the Baby Fae case about the possibility of using chimpanzee livers for some of our very tiny biliary atresia patients for who we could not find organs at that time. The rather extensive dialogue with people at the NIH escalated to the Director and eventually it came to the Ethics Committee of that agency. The proposal was shelved by mutual agreement. By this time the Baby Fae case had come up quite unexpectedly. We realized what a firestorm of publicity and of condemnation further heterograft trials were apt to bring down on us. I was stunned when I saw the reaction to the Baby Fae case. In the earlier trials (mine and all of Reemtsma's) . . . there was no particular sense of outrage. These earlier trials were not secret. Perhaps, the climate was different.

"If we could have helped our patients, the prospect of receiving abuse would not have been a deterrent. There was another factor and that was a White paper, issued by the NIH, at the end of a 5-year study. The conclusion published in Science was that only between 25 and 50 chimpanzees per year would be available in the United States for all of biomedical research, including that in the important fields of hepatitis and AIDS. The use of chimpanzees would further jeopardize an already endangered species, but without having an impact on the organ shortfall. We dropped the matter and have done nothing with it since."

After the Arden House conference, clinical xenotransplantation went into hibernation. Starzl, not one to give up easily, did make two more attempts in 1992–1993, when he and his team transplanted baboon livers into two patients, but after they failed even he put his efforts on hold. One thing was for certain—primates were out as donors. The gaze of the field had shifted to a different source for organs—pigs.

3 THE SCIENCE: DEFINING THE STEPS OF THE EVOLUTIONARY LADDER (1980–1991)

It took almost no imagination to hypothesize that chimpanzee organs could function in human recipients. Those advanced primates look like us, walk like us, and love like us. It is entirely radical to think the same thing about pig organs. To propose this and not be faced with laughter and mockery, scientists would need to develop a deep understanding of the differences between these two disparate species. What were the genetic variations that manifested over the millions of years of evolutionary selection that separated us from these animals that walk on four legs and enjoy rolling in the mud to cool off? Just describing these physiologic differences wouldn't be enough to excite anyone in a position to fund xenotransplantation. Basic strategies would need to be proposed and tested that could serve as a proof of principle that the organs from farm animals could function in humans.

While the Arden House meeting signaled the end of primate xenotransplantation, this hardly deterred the true believers in xeno, who had suspected for years that primates would be limited as a source of organs for transplant. The simplest reason for this was that primate organs were too small, as highlighted by James Hardy's failed attempt using the chimpanzee heart in 1964. There actually had been a few isolated attempts at transplanting pig, goat, and sheep organs into humans over the years, including one as early as 1906, but they failed rapidly.

Some of the earliest scientific work on xenotransplantation was conducted by Sir Roy Calne in London, one of the true fathers of transplantation and the person credited with the arrival of both azathioprine and cyclosporine into the clinic. In the era when Calne performed this work, in the 1950s and 1960s, transplantation was in its infancy, and the basic details of the immune system that seem obvious to us now were almost entirely unknown. These experiments, conducted between animals, served as much of a role in understanding basic transplant immunology as they did in informing the discipline of xenotransplantation.

In 1959, Calne transplanted a goat kidney into a dog and watched as it "underwent dramatic hyperacute rejection with hemorrhagic destruction within about 20 minutes, despite the main renal vessels being intact and patent." This was the first time Calne witnessed hyperacute rejection (meaning rapid rejection over minutes due to preformed antibodies that destroy the graft right after it is transplanted) with his own eyes, and he was able to confirm that it was due to pre-formed antibodies already present in the dog recipient. After Calne visited Reemtsma and Starzl when they were conducting their trials with chimpanzee and baboon kidneys in 1964, he convinced the chief veterinarian at the London Zoo to anesthetize a large baboon and bring him to the hospital where Calne was operating. "The baboon suddenly woke up, became alert, and looked exceedingly fierce, and it took a good deal of courage on the part of Dr. Graham-Jones to sedate it again. We hurriedly returned the baboon to the London zoo, and soon realized that the time was not right for transplants from animals to humans."[1]

Starting in 1968, Calne performed numerous liver transplants using pigs as donors and primates as recipients (including chimpanzees, baboons, Rhesus monkeys, and Cynomolgus monkeys). In some he used immunosuppression, and in some he didn't. Almost all of them died in a matter of hours, with one surviving three days before dying. He used livers because he knew this organ had an ability to survive the onslaught of antibodies much better than kidneys, and thought there was a chance the livers could withstand the dramatic hyperacute rejection. He conducted xenotransplant experiments using kidneys in pig-to-baboon and other disparate species with even worse results. Calne, the ultimate optimist when it came to progress in human transplantation, was pessimistic about the future of clinical xenotransplantation. He dabbled in the field thereafter but didn't devote significant energy or focus to it.

Another early series of experiments looking at the use of pig organs for transplant was published in 1966 by John Najarian.[2] Najarian was a transplant surgeon at University of California, San Francisco (UCSF) at the time, and would later become the chairperson of surgery at the University of Minnesota. He transplanted pig kidneys into dogs and dog kidneys into pigs. The pig-to-dog kidneys were rejected within ten to twenty minutes, while the dog-to-pig organs were lost in two to four hours. He confirmed that this rapid rejection was caused by pre-formed antibody that already existed in the recipient at the time of transplant. Despite utilizing numerous strategies including trying to absorb antibody out of the recipient blood, he could never prolong graft survival beyond a couple of hours.

While implantation of pig organs into humans were generally rare, the use of pig livers for ex-vivo perfusion (meaning hooking up a pig liver to the human blood vessels so that blood filters through the liver and returns to the human) was a different story. This was a reasonably common practice before liver transplantation was successful, with 141 attempts at pig perfusion of humans in liver failure in the 1960s and 1970s.[3] Most centers abandoned this practice once liver transplantation became a reality, as it was cumbersome and always unclear whether it really helped the patients.

In 1980, David Cooper, a freshly minted cardiac surgeon, showed up in Cape Town, South Africa with a burning interest in making xenotransplantation a reality.[4] South Africa seemed to be the perfect place to conduct this research. Baboons only cost twenty-five dollars, and few people were protesting the use of these animals in research. They were seemingly everywhere and considered a nuisance in daily life. As Cooper finished his clinical training in the United Kingdom in 1980, he reached out to Christian Barnard, the South African surgeon who had shocked the world when he performed the first human (-to-human) heart transplant on December 3, 1967, to ask if he had any space for a surgeon and researcher.

When Cooper arrived, he was keen to explore xenotransplantation, and he suggested it to his new mentor. Barnard responded that ". . . we have enough problems in preventing rejection of a human heart without taking on the added burden of a xenograft." Just three years prior, Barnard had attempted two xenotransplants into humans, neither of which worked. The first was a baboon heart, and the second a chimpanzee. They were placed heterotopically, as an auxiliary or second heart, with the patients' own hearts left in place. The two xenotransplants were performed in patients whose hearts had failed acutely after routine open heart surgery, and no human heart was immediately available to salvage them. The baboon heart recipient died six hours after the transplant, and the chimpanzee heart was rejected after four days leading to that patient's death. He lost interest in xenotransplant after that, telling Cooper "I became too attached to the chimpanzees."

Cooper was interested in exploring xeno in animal models, while Barnard was more of a "straight to human" kind of guy. But he was supportive of the work. Cooper started with transplants between African green (vervet) monkeys and baboons, to mimic the primate-to-human model. After a few years, it became clear to Cooper that while this line of research was important in understanding mechanisms of rejection and quantifying rejection in concordant species, it wouldn't ultimately be clinically applicable. He could read the writing on the wall earlier than most, that primates would not ultimately be the source of organs for humans. The problem wasn't related to immunological barriers—if it were, of course chimpanzees would be the donors of choice. But there were other challenges with primates. First, they were too difficult to breed. Second, other than chimpanzees, they were too small to be a reasonable source for human organs. Third, the risk of infection was too high, which the HIV pandemic (declared in 1981) made clear to anyone who wasn't already sure of this, as the virus originated in chimpanzees. Finally, the response to the Baby Fae case put the nail in the coffin. The public just wasn't going to support primate-to-human transplantation.

So in the early 1980s, Cooper turned his attention to pigs as potential donors. No one objected to breeding them for food, and if you could eat them, then it would be hard to protest their use in transplantation. Their litters were much larger than other similarly sized farm animals, and their organ size was also the most appropriate of all the farm animals. Cooper focused on the heterotopic heart model—sewing the pig heart into the abdomen of primates, so that it would contract after transplant and could be monitored by palpation and EKG tracings, but the heart didn't need to sustain the primate recipient's blood pressure and hemodynamics (and cardiopulmonary bypass wouldn't be required to perform the transplant).

Cooper performed a series of pig-to-baboon heterotopic heart transplants, and they all rejected violently and rapidly in minutes to hours. Pathology specimens confirmed that pre-formed antibody was to blame. Cooper didn't know what the antibodies were that were responsible for this rejection (what antigen they were binding to), but he figured if he could find a way to filter them out before transplant, perhaps he could prolong survival of these grafts. He designed a circuit to perfuse the recipient baboon blood through a pig kidney kept in a bowl outside the baboon for an hour or two or until the kidney turned black, with the filtered blood returning to the baboon. Then he followed this up with a pig-to-baboon heart transplant. This extended survival to four days. Cooper realized he would need a better understanding of what type of antibodies he was dealing with.

* * * * *

In 1983, Uri Galili had recently completed his PhD at Hebrew University in Jerusalem, and a post-doctoral fellowship at the famed Karolinska Institute in Stockholm.[5] He was now back in Israel working at the Hadassah Hospital in Jerusalem, studying how red blood cells in patients with blood diseases like beta-thalassemia get destroyed, leading to life-threatening anemia (low blood counts). He knew there were some surface abnormalities of these red blood cells, and as he examined them, he found that these cells extracted from human patients were bound with hundreds of antibodies on their surface. This was not true with normal healthy red blood cells. He noted that these antibodies could be coaxed to fall off the red blood cells when he mixed them with galactose (a type of sugar), but not other sugars or substances. He next looked at red blood cells from patients with sickle cell disease, and young and old red blood cells from healthy patients. These same antibodies were bound to the sickle cells, and older, senescent (aged and deteriorated) cells from healthy patients. Galili was able to identify which red blood cells were showing signs of senescence based on their biochemical characteristics.

In general, they were over 120 days old and would soon be cleared from the circulation. When he compared these cells to cells from the same patients that did not have senescence, those older cells had antibodies bound to them, whereas the younger, healthier cells did not.

Galili next passed the serum from normal patients of all blood types (the serum contains antibodies and other proteins, not cells) over columns with alpha-galactose coated onto them, and found that a full 1 percent of the antibodies present in the serum bound the columns. That was a much bigger proportion of antibodies than anyone would have expected (1 percent is a lot—in fact, this is the most abundant natural antibody in humans.). Those same antibodies strongly bound red blood cells from rabbits, which were known to carry alpha-galactose on their surface. He termed this natural (meaning it is present in every human, without a need for previous exposure) antibody "anti-alpha-galactosyl antibody," later to be known as "Alpha Gal antibody" (sometimes called anti-Gal, but we will stick with Alpha Gal antibody). Another important discovery that Galili reported in 1988 is that the Alpha Gal antibody binds multiple bacteria found commonly in the human gut microbiome, which likely explained why humans continue to make this antibody "naturally" at high levels throughout their lives—as a response to bacteria that live in all of our gut microbiomes.

By the mid-1980s, Galili had Alpha Gal antibody and its target Alpha Gal well characterized, but he was intrigued by the idea that humans had this natural antibody, but rabbits did not. Instead, the rabbits had the Alpha Gal sugar on a majority of their cells and secreted proteins. He and others began to characterize multiple animals, and discovered that mice, cows, pigs, dogs, rats, and rabbits all displayed Alpha Gal on their cells and lacked Alpha Gal antibody. He obtained blood from primates located at the San Francisco Zoo and found that apes and Old World monkeys (those from Asia and Africa) had Alpha Gal antibody and no Alpha Gal on their cells (like humans), whereas lemurs were like rabbits, with Alpha Gal on their cells and no Alpha Gal antibody in their serum. The gene that generated the enzyme that synthesized Alpha Gal was identified, and Gallili documented the presence of this enzyme in those animals that displayed Alpha Gal but not in humans. By 1991, the gene for this enzyme was identified in mouse and cow cells, and another group found that the same gene was present in humans but had a single-base deletion that stopped the production of Alpha Gal. They found similar deletions in apes and rhesus monkeys.[6]

All of these findings, combined with what was known of the evolution of Old World primates and New World primates, suggested that the gene was inactivated between 20 and 28 million years ago. The presumption is that there was a catastrophic pandemic caused by a pathogen (viral, bacterial, or otherwise) expressing Alpha Gal on its cell surfaces. Those primates that didn't express Alpha Gal antibody died in vast numbers, and those that had the mutation in the enzyme, leading to loss of the protein and generation of the antibody, were protected. The New World monkeys, that at this point had migrated to South America and were fully isolated from Old World monkeys, were not exposed to this pandemic. As humans evolved from primates many millions of years later, we maintained this genetic mutation in the Alpha Gal gene, and continue to be exposed to the Alpha Gal epitope in our gut microbiome, leading to sustained generation of antibody against Alpha Gal.

＊ ＊ ＊ ＊ ＊

In 1987, as Galili was characterizing the alpha Gal epitope and its natural antibody, Cooper moved to Baptist Medical Center in Oklahoma City. Cooper was recruited there to help start a cardiac transplant program. Ever since the approval of cyclosporine and dramatically improved outcomes with human allotransplantation, transplant programs were popping up around the country and transplant wait lists were growing exponentially, outstripping availability of human organs for transplant. Cooper, like transplant surgeons all across the world, was becoming increasingly frustrated caring for numerous heart-failure patients that he knew would never get organs in time.

At the same time, given his optimistic nature, he was more convinced than ever that the solution for his patients would require an unlimited source of organs, and it was more and more clear to him that the source would be pigs. The outcomes in animal models had shown that it wasn't time to move into human trials of xenotransplantation, as the science would need to be better defined in pre-clinical models first. He remained focused on the pig-to-primate model, but knew he needed to identify the antigen that was the target for natural antibodies leading to rapid rejection. His group had a simple idea to explore this. They perfused human plasma through the pig organs outside the body, as the organs sat in a sterile bowl. They then used some standard assays to collect the antibodies that had attached to the cells in the pig blood vessels, and sent them to a company for analysis. The company representative responded quite quickly and said the majority of the antibody was bound to Alpha Gal. That same company had a collaboration with Galili and was quite familiar with this target. This was the first time Alpha Gal was identified as the target for rapid rejection in xenotransplantation.

* * * * *

Just around the time Cooper was making his move to Oklahoma, a famous transplant researcher in London was becoming interested in snake venom. David White was a legend in the transplant field by this point, ten years removed from when he first convinced Sir Roy to try cyclosporine in a large animal model of transplantation. It had been White who performed the initial experiments with cyclosporine in rodents, while serving as the principal investigator in Sir Roy's lab. When he first presented the data to Calne showing essentially indefinite survival of transplants in these small animals, Calne didn't believe him and made him repeat the experiments again. Neither of them could have predicted the massive, world-changing effect the discovery and approval of cyclosporine would have on the discipline of transplant.[7]

At this point, White wasn't interested in xenotransplantation. He was too busy establishing himself as a principal investigator of his own lab, separate from the famous Sir Roy. He had just recently been appointed to a tenured position at the University of Cambridge in transplantation immunology, and was aiming to investigate more practical things. He saw xenotransplantation as a pipe dream. Despite his incredulity, White did collaborate with a colleague on a small project transplanting rabbit kidneys into pigs. They were able to prevent hyperacute rejection by using cobra venom factor. To understand this better, a bit of background on antibodies is required.

The concept of antibodies protecting against infection was first described in 1890, when researchers identified that the transfer of serum from animals immunized to diphtheria could cure different animals infected with the bacteria. Shortly thereafter, in 1900, Paul Ehrlich proposed that a protein he termed "antibodies" are present in the serum. He identified that antibodies were branched structures that had multiple sites that could bind to foreign material, known as "antigen." Ehrlich further described the complement system. He was experimenting with the ability of antibodies in serum to bind and lyse bacteria and blood cells. He identified a separate protein in the serum that "complemented" the effects of antibodies and led to the lysis of the bacteria and blood cells.[8]

It's worth digging a bit deeper into the complement system, as it will play a major role in xenotransplant rejection.[9] Complement doesn't just sit in the serum, waiting for antibody to find a target so it can pounce and unleash its destructive properties. Complement is found in an inactive state, and is activated when antibody binds to antigen. The bound entity forms an immune complex, which then initiates the complement cascade that leads to the formation of a membrane attack complex, which can blow holes through bacteria, viruses, dying cells, and healthy cells as well. The system is highly regulated with complement regulatory proteins that can halt complement activation when it's going too far or occurring where it shouldn't be. These regulatory proteins are critical, and patients who have dysfunctional regulatory proteins often also have severe autoimmune diseases. As an additional safety factor, many of the complement proteins degrade rather quickly, further limiting the length and strength of the complement response. A component in snake venom (cobra venom factor or CVF) has long been known to first activate, but then rapidly deplete, complement, leading to inactivation of this pathway.[10] Complement is a critical arm of the immune system, with the concentration of complement exceeding the amount of immunoglobulin (antibody) in the serum of humans. It is required for so many of the immune system functions, and yet we rarely talk about it in health care. The above discussion is more than most clinicians remember about the function of complement.

In 1987, White and colleagues reported on their ability to prolong the survival of rabbit kidney grafts that were transplanted into pigs using CVF.[11] It was published in a pretty minor journal, and he really didn't think much of it. White was no more interested in complement than anyone else he knew in healthcare. When he was approached by a well-known cardiac surgeon by the name of John Wallwork who wanted to talk to him about a potential project, White figured it would be one of those annoying meetings with a clinician who had no idea what it was he wanted to do in the lab. Little did White know this meeting would lead to a collaboration that would change the trajectory of his entire career.

* * * * *

John Wallwork was frustrated that a patient of his had just died waiting for a heart transplant.[12] This wasn't a one-time occurrence for Wallwork. After the approval of cyclosporine a few years before, heart transplantation became a reality overnight, with one-year survival after transplant better than 90 percent. As exciting as that was, the list of patients needing transplants rapidly expanded, but the availability of hearts did not. Wallwork found himself caring for patients every day that were near death's door, and he knew most of them would die. He had seen White's paper on the rabbits and the pigs, and was excited when he realized that White was working at his same institution. Shortly after the death of his latest waitlisted patient, Wallwork came to White's office and asked him why he couldn't have just put a pig heart into his patient. Maybe it could have worked temporary, to bridge him to a human heart? White explained that it would have been hyperacutely rejected, as humans have pre-formed antibodies to pigs. Wallwork countered that he found that unlikely. His patient was Jewish, so how could he have antibodies against pigs?

Despite the rather limited data on the potential success of complement depletion, Wallwork was convinced this line of research warranted serious consideration. He convinced White to join him and a local businessman in setting up a company with the goal of making xenotransplantation a clinical reality. The company would be named Imutran. Wallwork went off to America to drum up some funding for the lab, and somehow succeeded. He convinced someone at the financial firm Warburg Pincus to invest in Imutran. Wallwork was the ultimate optimist, a rather colorful character, and he never took no for an answer.

A scientific advisory board for Imutran was established, which included some prominent scientists in London, including the person who invented monoclonal antibodies. They shared spirited discussions about the most significant barriers to successful xenotransplantation. Some were convinced that it was all about the preformed antibodies—get rid of those and the rest of the immune response could be controlled with cyclosporine. Others believed the antibodies were really just the tip of the iceberg. They predicted that even if the antibody response was negated, a violent cellular-mediated rejection would ensue that would destroy the graft. White fell in the antibody camp, but he had to prove it. He did a little thinking, and quickly came up with a strategy that he knew would give him an answer about whether antibody was necessary to cause rapid rejection in a xenotransplant.[13]

White was aware that piglets are born without antibodies, as antibodies don't cross the placenta in pigs. Piglets typically receive antibodies from the colostrum of the mother, until they eventually begin making their own after a few months. So, if he could separate newborn piglets from their mothers and transplant them with rabbit kidneys, those piglets wouldn't have antibodies and thus wouldn't hyperacutely reject the grafts. Then after a few days, he could start feeding the pigs porcine colostrum, and watch the grafts rapidly reject. He would further be able to remove the grafts at different time points and identify exactly what the antibody was that was destroying the graft.

The experiment proved more challenging than he expected but after working through some roadblocks, he finally succeeded in performing the transplants, and much to his surprise they rapidly rejected. Examination under the microscope confirmed that the destroyed grafts had no evidence of antibody deposition. He discovered that the grafts were absolutely coated in complement. White repeated the experiment, and showed that if he pretreated the piglets with cobra venom factor, hyperacute rejection was prevented. So maybe in the end dealing with antibody wasn't needed.

Strong debate among the advisory board followed. Why had complement caused hyperacute rejection of the rabbit grafts without antibody? Despite the deep understanding of immunology that was present in that board, complement was not anyone's focus. White and his colleagues read everything there was to know about complement and discovered that all cells in humans and animals display regulatory proteins on their surface that prevent activation of and lysis by the complement system. These regulatory proteins, termed Complement Regulatory Proteins (CRP), act as a shield, or maybe more as a password that the cells can give to circulating complement, to prevent activation of the complement cascade and assured destruction that would surely follow. After much debate, the advisory board decided White needed to generate a pig that expressed human CRPs that would prevent the activation of complement. They figured it had to be human so that it would work in the eventual intended recipient.

Before trying to make a genetically modified pig, White set out to generate a mouse that expressed human regulatory proteins. Although White had never made a transgenic animal before, the technique of injecting purified DNA into a fertilized mouse oocyte (egg) had been described in 1980, and researchers at the University of Cambridge, White's institution, were well versed in the protocol.[14] White first treated female mice with hormones obtained from a pregnant horse (gonadotropin), followed by human gonadotropin. Then these female mice were housed with male mice overnight. Mating ensued, and the next day the fertilized mice were sacrificed, and their ovaries removed. The fertilized oocytes were harvested and placed in a dish under a microscope. Fifty tiny eggs were sucked up in a small syringe and placed in an injection chamber. Then, White injected the DNA for his cloned regulatory protein right into the nuclei of the oocytes.

Next, White obtained some female mice that had been mated to male mice that had undergone vasectomies. This caused them to be pseudopregnant. This is a similar state to being pregnant, only without the presence of a fetus. It occurs in certain mammals (cats, dogs, pigs, rats, and mice), although not humans, after copulation with an infertile male. After that mating the corpus luteum (an ovulated follicle) persists even without an embryo, leading to progesterone hormone secretion, mammary gland generation, lactation, and maternal behavior (like building nests). By generating pseudopregnant mice in the lab, White had surrogates that could develop his fertilized fetuses into mice. These pseudopregnant mice were anesthetized, and their bellies opened. Their ovaries, oviducts, and uteri were identified, and twenty-five fertilized and genetically modified eggs were injected into the oviduct leading into the uterus. The mice were sewn shut and recovered.

To add to the technical difficulty of this, in a majority of cases, the transfected gene doesn't incorporate into the nucleus and the gene isn't expressed. Mice have a gestation period of three weeks and an average of six pups in each litter. The pups stay with the mother for another three to four weeks until they can be weaned. Once they are weaned, a small piece of the tail from the baby mouse can be clipped and genetic analysis is done to see if the gene is expressed. If it is expressed, then three to four more weeks are required until that mouse is ready for breeding, to expand the mice available for testing. This adds up to nine to eleven weeks from the time of injecting the DNA until breeding of the transgenic animals can commence. The yield on incorporation of DNA and expression in the mice is on order of 1 percent using this technique.[15]

This was not a project for the faint of heart. But White approached it with vigor and persistence. He successfully generated mice with a few different human regulatory proteins. He perfused their tiny kidneys with human blood, and showed that complement was not deposited. Most importantly, he learned how to make transgenic animals, and proved, at least to himself, that it could be done with these particular regulatory proteins. He was ready to move on to the pig.

* * * * *

In addition to David Cooper and David White, there was another brilliant David who, in the 1970s, came to recognize that the pig would become the donor of choice for xenotransplantation. David Howard Sachs was born on January 10th, 1942, at 2:38 p.m. in a Manhattan hospital. His father ran a jewelry store in Brooklyn, and his mother stayed home and raised him along with his older brother and younger sister. Sachs was a happy and curious baby and toddler until 1946, when he was four and a half years old. It all started with a fever and headache, but when he suddenly couldn't move his left leg, Sachs's parents knew something was wrong. He was diagnosed with paralytic polio, one of the most feared diseases in the world. He was admitted to Manhattan's Hospital for Special Surgery, where he then began a year of procedures, therapy, and isolation from other children. Sachs has strong memories of his time in the hospital, and in particular the painful spinal taps he repeatedly endured.

Sachs was told he may never walk again—but even at the tender age of four, he knew that would not be the case. "It just never seemed possible to me that I wouldn't. It just seemed to me that I had to get over this problem. I've never had a defeatist attitude toward anything. I always feel that it's just a matter of being able to figure it out, make it work. That's my attitude toward everything."[16]

Sachs spent a year with a physical therapist learning how to walk again, utilizing the still-working muscles in his atrophied left leg and foot. He mastered it perfectly, and to this day most people aren't even aware that he ever had this illness. "My feet are two different sizes. I buy two different sets of shoes and have to split them. You wouldn't know it unless I told you, but they're different."[17] If you were trying to trace the origins of Sachs's self-reliance, resilience, and belief in success against all odds, this childhood illness might be it.

Sachs was precocious and brilliant, acing every class he ever took without putting in much effort. He developed a love of all things mechanical, fixing things around the house and rebuilding car engines. He also discovered a lifelong love of gardening. "Still today when I see a seedling come up it just gives me a feeling of excitement. Every time I've moved to a new house the first thing I've done is gone out back and figured out where I was going to have my vegetable garden, and turned over the soil and planted my seeds. I just love gardening—every spring to see the renewal."[18]

As Sachs was nearing college, he was already considering a career in medicine, driven by his love of problem solving, a desire to live up to his nickname "Mr. Fix-it," and of course his own experiences with illness as a child. Sachs majored in chemistry at Harvard, graduating *summa cum laude* in 1963. He then went on to do a Fulbright fellowship in Paris in organic chemistry. It was there that he realized that he loved Paris, loved learning foreign languages (he speaks five), and didn't want a career in chemistry. He entered Harvard Medical School in 1964, where his interest quickly turned to surgery. He had early exposure to the field of transplantation. Sachs was fascinated in particular by the accomplishments of Peter Medawar, the English immunologist who won the Nobel Prize in 1960. It was in Sachs's second year of medical school that he heard a lecture describing Medawar's finding that dizygotic cows (twins that came from two eggs, or are fraternal rather than identical) that shared a placenta could accept skin grafts from each other without immunosuppression. They were tolerant to these grafts because they were chimeric—they had stem cells from each other that were long-lived and prevented immune responses against each other. (This is not true in humans, where dizygotic or fraternal twins tend to have separate placentas and no mixing of stem cells, making them no more genetically related than any other type of siblings).

Medawar followed up this observation by injecting cells from unrelated rabbits into rabbit embryos in utero. After birth, Medawar transplanted skin from rabbits matched to the cell donor onto these chimeric recipients, and the skin was accepted without immunosuppression. This was the first example of tolerance in a living animal, and the first time a transplant was successful between two non-identical animals, published in 1953.[19] Sachs knew right then and there that this would be part of his life's work. "It just blew my mind," Sachs said. "The possibility of being able to give people a new life when they're dying because an organ is failing—and doing it without having to give them drugs that could kill them—it just seemed to me that this was very important."

There was another thing, maybe just as important. Sachs knew he could figure it out. It might take a while, but he knew it was possible because it had already been shown to work. Sachs always believed that anything that was displayed in nature in some form could be understood and then applied in another setting. "Tolerance in conventional transplantation, he had decided, was solvable." Sachs summarized his philosophy years later when delivering a speech accepting the Medawar Prize, the premier prize in transplantation research, fittingly named after the man whose work inspired him to enter the field in the first place. "For me, experiments of nature have always provided the most important proof of principle for the validity of unexpected biological phenomena."[20]

Sachs graduated from medical school in 1968 and began his surgical residency. It was then that he read everything that had been published on transplantation and transplant immunology. He next turned his attention to xenotransplantation. He read about Reemtsma's transplants with chimpanzees, conducted just four years earlier. The knowledge that one of the chimpanzee kidney transplants worked for more than nine months in a human convinced Sachs that he was witnessing another example of nature showing the way. "I already had the idea that we were going to need another source of organs besides humans, that the need for organs was going to exceed the availability of donors. I saw no reason why the organ of an animal—other than the brain—would not be as good an organ as the organ of a human being."

Sachs completed two years of his surgical residency at Massachusetts General Hospital and then went into the lab for a planned two-year research fellowship. He found a spot at the National Institutes of Health (NIH) in Bethesda, Maryland in 1970. His research progressed so rapidly that after just two years he was offered his own lab at the NIH. It was an offer he couldn't pass up. Sachs applied for an extension of his leave of absence from residency, which was granted. In the next two years, he would achieve one of the most important discoveries of his career, identifying a major portion of the immune system that had not been previously recognized—the Major Histocompatibility Complex (MHC) Class II.[21] This family of proteins, along with those in the MHC Class I, plays a central role in organ rejection.[22] The variability of these proteins between individuals is what allows us to fight off novel viruses and bacteria, as each of us expresses different MHC proteins. Because of this, the odds that a single virus or other pathogen can kill off an entire population is reduced. The different variations of the MHC allow our immune system to recognize self from non-self, allowing destruction of bacteria, viruses, and cancers, but avoiding autoimmune responses to self-proteins. Unfortunately, it is this same variability that causes us to reject organs from donors that are not identical to us. We didn't evolve to be able to accept organ transplants from each other.

This discovery earned Sachs admission into the upper echelon of immunology researchers. By 1974, he was appointed chief of the Transplantation

Biology Section in the Immunology Branch at the NIH. He still harbored dreams of returning to his surgery residency, and continued to apply for extensions to his research leave from the hospital. He jokes to this day that he is the oldest active surgery resident in the world.

Now that Sachs had a big discovery under his belt, he felt liberated to conduct some cutting-edge, aspirational research. Ever since he read about Reemtsma's results from transplants with chimpanzees conducted a decade before, he believed xenotransplantation was something he could solve. Sachs knew, even in the 1970s, that primates were never going to be the donor of choice. Chimpanzees would never be accepted as donors, given their endangered status and their behavior that so closely resembled our own. Baboons were too small, bred slowly, and had one baby at a time (meaning it would be slow and expensive to generate a herd, and even more difficult to consider in-breeding strategies or eventually gene therapy), and also carried the potential risk of disease transmission. Sachs theorized that an animal that humans interacted with for food and farming would be ideal, since the risk of a novel infection jumping into humans would be low. But most farm animals, including horses, cows, and outbred pigs were too big to be organ donors to humans.

One day in the early 1970s, Sachs was visiting the NIH animal facility, and the manager there asked him if he had ever heard of miniature swine. These were pigs that had escaped into the wilderness and lived on what food they could find. Over many hundreds of years, they underwent natural selection for smaller size, requiring less sustenance. Sachs began researching them and found characteristics he liked—organs that were similar in size to those of adult humans, sexual maturity at five months, females that were fertile every three weeks and had a gestation period of under four months, and litter sizes that could reach ten piglets. He knew immediately what this meant. He could breed them for their MHCs. He would use his antibodies that identified the MHC Class I and II to classify which MHC the pigs had. He then would select out those pigs that had similar MHCs and breed them together, eventually achieving strains that were homozygous (the same genetically) for Class I, Class II, or both. This would allow him to use these pigs as donors in transplant experiments, and select the immunologic barrier he was crossing in any transplant. Without this type of defined herd, every transplant would be across a random and un-repeatable mismatch that could lead to more or less stringent rejection.

It took him a few years, but once he accomplished this, he was the only person in the world who had a large animal herd allowing for transplants across specified immunologic mismatches. This proved to be critical for establishing tolerance protocols that allowed transplants between animals without long-term immunosuppression, protocols he then successfully moved into primates and eventually humans. It also has helped him over the years in his xeno experiments; Sachs was always convinced that the only way to successfully conduct xenotransplant into man was to make a human tolerant to a pig organ. Otherwise, he theorized, too much immunosuppression will be required.

While Sachs was working on establishing his pig herd, he spent the next twenty years performing various transplants in mice and rats. The bulk of his work was focused on models of tolerance, using techniques that would be realistic to translate into humans. His work boiled down to two main strategies. The first, borrowed directly from the work of Medawar, was to transfer bone marrow from a donor while simultaneously giving immunosuppression, to allow engraftment of those cells. The immunosuppressive regimen was tailored to allow engraftment but not destroy all of the recipient cells, establishing a state of "mixed chimerism," which means donor and host bone marrow cells (termed hematopoietic cells) both exist in the host.[23]

The second strategy involved the thymus, a critical organ of the immune system that sits in the chest in front of the heart and is most active in the first few years of life in humans, involuting or shrinking down by our teenage years.[24] Consider the thymus as T Cell University. Immature T cells are generated in the bone marrow before they migrate to the thymus to undergo maturation or education at the university.[25] These immature T cells have untested T cell receptors on their surface, but as these receptors form, an error-prone process of gene rearrangements allows numerous different potential receptors to result, some of which may work well and some of which may be faulty.

Once the immature T cells arrive in the thymus, at the university, they enroll in two major courses—positive selection and negative selection. In positive selection, which takes place in the cortex or outer portion of the thymus, immature T cells bind to MHC Class I or Class II molecules on cells that line the cortex. If these immature cells fail to bind (the T cell receptor is faulty), they are destroyed. If they bind well to MHC class I, they become CD 8+ T cells. If they bind well to MHC class II, they become CD 4+ T cells. Both CD 8+ and CD 4+ T cells function and overlap in our immune system, but their roles are distinct. CD8+ cells, sometimes called killer T cells, have direct killing mechanisms. Once they have been activated by other immune cells, they can bind directly to targets on other cells that contain bacteria, viruses, or have become cancers, and directly kill these cells. CD 4+ cells, sometimes called helper T cells, play a central role in activating and enhancing an immune response. Once these cells themselves are activated by a specific antigen, they release cytokines (or cellular messengers) to attract other immune cells, including CD8+ T cells. They also attract and activate B cells, leading to antibody production that is specific to a particular antigen.

These somewhat mature T cells now move on to the medulla of the thymus, where they undergo negative selection. In this demanding advanced course, these cells are presented self-proteins in the MHC groove. If they bind tightly to these self-proteins, they are destroyed to prevent autoimmunity. Roughly 98 percent of immature T cells fail to graduate T Cell University and are destroyed, with only 2 percent exiting the thymus to become mature, functioning T cells. Talk about a rigorous university.

As Sachs and his team learned more about the thymus and its potential role in rejection, they realized that when they added direct thymic irradiation to their bone marrow transplant protocol, the thymus was repopulated with cells from the transplanted and recipient bone marrow. In this newly chimeric thymus, maturing cells would then undergo positive and negative selection. Cells that reacted to either the host or the donor cells were destroyed in this repopulated thymus, leading to long-term stable mixed chimerism. In other words, cells from both the host and the donor became teachers in the thymus, both giving the course on negative selection.

Once mixed chimerism was established, with transplanted bone marrow and native bone marrow existing in harmony, a skin graft could be transplanted from the same animal as the bone marrow donor without immunosuppression. The animal was tolerant to that particular organ with a functioning immune system to other insults. They were then able to extend this protocol to his inbred miniature swine, with some adjustments, and make these pigs tolerant to kidney and heart transplants. His success in these large animals depended on his ability to choose the MHC mismatch he wanted to test, something he was able to do because of the breeding strategy he employed since his early days at NIH.

In 1991, Sachs was invited back to Massachusetts General Hospital (MGH). He became a professor in the Department of Surgery, even while still officially on leave from his surgical residency. He would run a large animal research lab, working with his herd of pigs (he had more than four hundred by this point), which would be transferred to a farm in rural Massachusetts, a less than two-hour drive from Boston. He would also have facilities for monkeys, to conduct pre-clinical work in a relevant animal model. Sachs was excited to be part of a busy clinical transplant program, where he would have the opportunity to translate his findings into the clinic. He would spend one day per week rounding on the inpatient transplant service at the hospital. One of the first things he did upon arriving at MGH as director of the newly formed Transplantation Biology Research Center (TBRC) was recruit Megan Sykes, a hematologist (physician who studies blood diseases) who had worked in his lab at the NIH and was central to his discoveries there. Dr. Sykes quickly developed a laboratory focusing on mechanisms of tolerance in mouse models of transplant and xenotransplant, while Sachs turned his focus to large animal models. He was ready to finally sink his teeth into the xeno world.

4 THE POTENTIAL: THE COMMODIFICATION OF XENO (1991–2004)

The 1990s represented a golden age for xenotransplantation. Although gene editing was in its infancy, the idea that designer pigs could be generated to serve as bespoke organs for anyone in need captured the imagination of scientists, the press, and the industry titans who wrote big checks looking for even bigger payouts. The sense that clinical transplantation was right around the corner was palpable, magnified by one of the biggest scientific advances of the last century—the ability to clone a living large animal. This era was when it became clear that xenotransplantation could lead to a major financial payoff, and that the engineered pigs themselves would be the commodity that would unlock this windfall. Industry leaders wanted to hold that key. All it would take was some brilliant, persistent minds, cutting-edge science, and a lot of money.

———

It was the early 1990s. David White's entire lab effort was focused on the work of Imutran, with the goal of making xenotransplantation a reality. The endeavor of making transgenic pigs was on an entirely different scale than generating mice. A pig facility needed to be built, adhering to specific onerous regulatory requirements to eventually allow their organs to be used in humans. They needed lab space, an operating theater, and multiple experienced staff members. They needed money.

The most common route for funding a basic science lab is through basic science grants sponsored and paid for by the government. In the United Kingdom, the national funding agency is the UK Research and Innovation (UKRI) agency, and in the United States it is the National Institutes of

Health (NIH). A researcher who has a project or line of research will submit a comprehensive grant that goes through a complex process of peer review and if the science is deemed worthy, the grant may be selected for funding. These grants are quite competitive, with pay lines in the tenth to fifteenth percentile (meaning 85–90 percent of submitted grants get rejected). In general, funding is reserved for scientific endeavors that focus on mechanisms of science (how something works) rather than on scaling up a particular treatment for a disease, and are on the order of hundreds of thousands of dollars per year of funding. This is typically enough money to do some specific experiments, but not enough to perform a major clinical trial or bring a product to the market. In order to translate laboratory discoveries into actual treatments for disease, forming a company with industry support is often the most realistic option, as larger sums of money are required in a much shorter time frame than the government agencies can respond. It typically takes a year or more to obtain funding from the NIH once an application for funding is submitted.

White went on a world tour, talking to investors on both sides of the pond. His witty personality and ability to simplify the most complex mechanisms of the immune system served him well. His slide deck included humorous cartoons that denoted complement as a bomb. He then described his genetic modifications as a strategy of flying under the radar, avoiding the friendly fire of complement. His pictures included caricatures of British troops in World War II, complete with British flags and funny faces.

White was a hit, and for years afterwards he was asked to share his slides in the transplant community. He raised the necessary money. One of the early investors, the company Sandoz, was a major supporter of White from the days of the discovery of cyclosporine. It didn't hurt that one of Imutran's advisors was none other than Roy Calne. Between the two of them, White and Calne had helped the pharmaceutical company earn billions of dollars on cyclosporine. Evidently, it seemed worth taking a chance with White again.

With money in hand, White and his group focused on making transgenic pigs. The process was very similar to the techniques used in mice. Female pigs were injected with hormones to make them hyperovulate. One day later, they were mated with a boar. A day after that, the fertilized eggs, or embryos, were removed from these pregnant sows under anesthesia. The cloned DNA for the human complement regulatory protein Decay Accelerating Factor (DAF) was then injected into the nuclei of the embryos, and then twenty-five of those injected embryos were gathered for implantation in each surrogate sow. The surrogate sows, similar to the mice, were mated with vasectomized boars, becoming pseudopregnant. The twenty-five embryos were carefully implanted in the uteri of these surrogates, and pregnancy ensued. Then White and his team would wait roughly four months until the transgenic piglets would be ready for delivery.

It is worth reviewing some of the challenges of this process. When you inject a small amount of DNA into an embryo, its integration into the DNA of the fertilized egg is random. It can go anywhere, can silence other important genes, and may not be associated with any promoter region, so it may or may not be expressed (and expression level can be low). Less than 5 percent of the embryos that have been injected with the cloned DNA will go on to express the gene of interest in their cells. One top of that, only 10 to 20 percent of implanted embryos will develop and be born as piglets. So if twenty-five injected embryos are implanted in the surrogate sow, perhaps only one of them will actually have the ability to express the gene, and only two to five of the injected embryos will be born as a viable piglet. You would be lucky to get a single piglet that is born that expresses a gene. These are the kind of odds you are up against.

Once the piglets are born, they are genotyped to look for expression of the gene, in this case DAF. If they express the gene, then they will be used for breeding. For a male or female pig, you have to wait about six months before they are ready for breeding. The male offers some advantages, as it can be bred with multiple sows. As we generally get genes from each of our parents, if you breed a male and female pig that both express the gene of interest (and are homozygous for it, meaning both copies of that gene are present), then the offspring will also express the gene. Some transgenic animals breed poorly, and in these cases you have to breed animals that are heterozygous for the gene of interest (or have one copy of the gene of interest from one parent, but are negative for it from the other parent). When heterozygous animals are bred, only 25 percent of the litter will be homozygous for the gene of interest. We are really talking a year for a transgenic animal to be generated, matured, bred, and for the next generation of piglets born. That's assuming any of the transgenic animals actually express the gene of interest.

Nevertheless, in less than two years, White succeeded. He summarized the experience in his humble and disarming demeanor: "I am sure I was involved in the process, but I can take no credit for the fact that all this was accomplished in a remarkably short time. A contribution that I can recollect is that just before Christmas of 1992 I acted as the midwife for the birth of our first litter of pigs, which by random chance included one transgenic pig whom we called Astrid. Pigs do not need really need a midwife; I was only there so I could later claim to have been present."[1] While Astrid was born sometime before Christmas, the press jumped on the idea that she was born on Christmas Eve. White, understanding the importance of creating a legend, did little to dispel this. "At a secret location in Cambridgeshire, researchers inject human DNA into a pig embryo. Six months later Astrid, the world's first transgenic pig, is born—of a virgin, in a sterile stable, on Christmas eve."[2]

Astrid was just the start. One animal was great, but they would need many more to conduct any real experiments. Over the next eighteen months, through this process of pronuclear injection and breeding, White's group generated seventy-nine different lines of pigs transgenic for DAF.[3] "Acting on the principle that 'more is better,' we selected a couple of very high-expressing pigs from which to breed and test as organ donors."

"The 5 years between 1993 and 1997 were a whirlwind of testing and documenting resistance to hyperacute rejection of various organs from these pigs. Overall, we published more than 80 papers, took part in a TV documentary, and held a press-conference that promptly stimulated the UK government to pass a law regulating clinical xenotransplantation—they set up a committee."[4]

Before White could start transplanting the transgenic pig organs into primates, he had to get approval from the United Kingdom's interior ministry, which regulates animal experiments in the country. In the meantime, he set up perfusion systems where pig organs would be perfused with human blood, and then the organs would be removed from the circuit and examined for the presence of antibody, complement, or signs of hyperacute rejection.

Finally, after *ex vivo* perfusion of every organ White could think of, and numerous publications, the Home Office finally (reluctantly) gave the go ahead for White and his team to begin transplants into primates. The first model they used was the heterotopic heart transplant, sewing hearts from pigs into the bellies of monkeys. In a first set of experiments that used no immunosuppression, the transgenic pig hearts had a median survival of five days, although none suffered hyperacute rejection.[5] In a second experiment where conventional immunosuppression including cyclosporine was given, the transgenic hDAF hearts beat for a median of forty days, whereas all the controls were lost to hyperacute rejection within hours. These results were met with serious excitement in the transplant community, and even more fanfare in the lay press. "Led by the brilliant Cambridge University immunologist David White and the heart surgeon John Wallwork, director of transplant surgery at Papworth hospital, they bred pigs that had been genetically modified to overcome the problem of rejection and provide a source of "farmed" organs for transplant into humans . . . The scientists could barely contain their excitement and, at a celebratory press conference, they said they expected to carry out the first human transplant within a couple of years."[6]

Not long after reporting the transgenic cardiac transplants, the team conducted kidney transplants into monkeys with the same immunosuppression. Survival was more modest, although the transgenic hDAF kidneys continued to avoid hyperacute rejection and outlast wild-type kidneys. The median survival of these life-sustaining kidneys (the recipients native kidneys were removed at the time of transplant) was thirteen days, with one surviving thirty-five days.[7] In a follow-up experiment, they would show that including a splenectomy at the time of transplant significantly improved survival of these modified kidneys, with half surviving fifty days and one lasting seventy-eight days.[8] (The spleen is an organ that is considered part of the immune system, serving as a super-powered lymph node with a role in cellular and antibody function, and activation of many immune responses depend on the presence of this organ.) This was a dramatic improvement compared to anything that had been accomplished without transgenic pigs.

These results were enough to impress one group of keen observers—the pharmaceutical industry. Sandoz had recently merged with Ciba-Geigy to form Novartis, one of the biggest companies in the world. They had money to burn and were ready to take a risk. They approached White and his team and made an offer they couldn't refuse. This move followed an analysis conducted by Salomon Brothers that detailed the "unrecognized potential of xenotransplantation," predicting a $6 billion market for transgenic organs by 2010.[9] The Novartis CEO, Daniel Vasella, announced he would spend a cool $1 billion on research, predicting mass-market transplantation of these organs by 2004. These optimistic reports were picked up by newspaper columnists around the country, who printed quotes predicting that "we might each have our own Astrids, 'self pigs' custom-made from our own DNA, 'immunological twins' available for any spare parts we might need in the course of our lives."[10]

Imutran was grabbing headlines and funding, and the purchase by Novartis was front-page news across the world. The infusion of money into the small company that had been subsisting on small investments and competitive grants was a welcome occurrence, but it did come with some strings. Novartis quickly brought in a medical director, a staff of immunologists, a pharmacology team, and a regulatory staff. White had his frustrations about working according to the protocols and schedules of a massive pharmaceutical company with the goal of bringing a "product" to market on an ambitious timeline. "Slowly, Novartis imposed protocol-driven R and D pathways used for drug development onto transgenic pigs." But White knew that what they really needed to be doing was continuing to create more transgenic pigs, and then breed them until they had herds to experiment with. He also believed they would need more than a "herd of Astrids." He wanted pigs that expressed all three known complement regulatory proteins. His frustration was captured in an interview with a local paper. "We can throw money at the problem till we're blue I the face, but pigs won't grow any quicker, not even if you feed them dollar bills."[11]

Novartis set up an international xenotransplant team, which included five major North American transplant centers. Their mandate was to develop a clinically applicable immunosuppressive regimen to be trialed with the transgenic pigs in a pig-to-primate model. This proved to be cumbersome, and it required multiple visits by White and his team to help get these protocols in motion. Imutran continued preclinical transplants into primates, but most of the work was moved to a private facility in the Netherlands. This required flying pigs and Cambridge surgeons to the facility, where they would conduct the transplants and then shuttle back home, leaving local Dutch veterinarians to take care of the animals.

White was spending the bulk of his time on the road, talking to collaborators, investors, the press, or sitting in boardrooms. He had almost no opportunity to camp out in his lab planning experiments and reviewing data, his true passion. He was actually quite gifted as a communicator, a true master at explaining difficult scientific concepts to people with backgrounds in finance and business, all while throwing in humor and charisma. But it wasn't what he wanted to be doing. Even more frustrating to him, he wasn't the one deciding on the experiments worth conducting. But the leadership at Novartis didn't want to spend time exploring different scientific strategies. They were aiming to move forward as quickly as possible, focusing on the ultimate goal—bringing their product to market. It wasn't driven solely by a desire to realize their investment as fast as possible. They weren't the only show in xeno-town. Formidable competition was breathing down their necks.

* * * * *

"The building sits at the end of a long gravel road on a slight knoll in the middle of a 200-acre lot in the little farming hamlet of Albany, Ohio. There are no signs outside, which is by design. 'We're not big on signs.' . . . On the rare occasion when uninvited guests drop in with nosy questions, a supervisor dismissed them with a simple, if less than completely truthful, explanation: 'We breed pigs.'[12]

These are the quotes of John Logan, who was the scientific director and executive at Nextran, a biotechnology company based in Princeton, New

Jersey that ran the Ohio pig-breeding facility. Like Imutran, Nextran began as a small outfit of a few scientists on a shoestring budget attempting to generate transgenic mice and swine with human regulatory proteins. Their strategy was quite similar to White's, who was a few years ahead of them. Nextran had a few unique angles—placing two or three complement regulatory proteins on each pig, and also throwing in a human sugar molecule that could potentially reduce the expression of Alpha Gal. They attracted interest from Baxter International, the medical products manufacturer. Baxter bought 70 percent of the company in 1994, changing the name to Nextran. It may seem strange that Baxter, a medical products company, would have interest in xenotransplantation. But a large portion or their business was in equipment for dialysis, and they were looking for an entrance into the transplant world.

At the same time that Imutran was plugging its transgenic organs into monkeys, Nextran's pig organs were being placed in baboons, primarily by surgeons at the Mayo Clinic. Although they were also able to avoid hyperacute rejection, their long-term survival was shorter than White's. This was one of the reasons Imutran was always leading the pack in the field of xenotransplantation. Another was presentation. White's team birthed Astrid in 1992. Nextran didn't start until a few years after that. Logan and his team used virtually the same process to generate and then breed transgenic pigs, a process Logan described as "horribly inefficient." In his experience, for every hundred eggs that his team injected with human genes and then implanted into a surrogate, twenty pigs would be born, but only one would have the gene of interest.

There was one area where Nextran was in the lead, though—in the field of liver perfusion. In 1997, after publication of their results with pig-to-baboon transplantation, Nextran obtained FDA approval to conduct a Phase 1 clinical trial of liver perfusion in patients who presented near death with failing livers. These pig livers would be used as a temporary bridge to transplant, using the same technique published previously by a team at Duke in 1994 (using wild-type pigs).[13] One of Nextran's centers was Baylor University Medical Center in Dallas. On September 3, 1997, some of Nextran's transgenic pigs were shipped to Baylor by truck. There they sat in the large animal lab, monitored by the research veterinarians who insured they were healthy and well cared for. Marlon Levy, the site investigator for the pig perfusion project, was searching everywhere for a patient.

On October 2, a man by the name of Robert Pennington would be the first human to be treated by a transgenic pig. Pennington was a healthy young man who lived with his grandparents and worked at the family-owned carpet store. He started to feel sick in early September. He didn't think much of it until one morning towards the end of the month he looked in the mirror and saw yellow eyes staring back at him. He went to a local clinic, but was sent home with instructions to follow up with a specialist. A few days later he worsened, becoming confused, lethargic, and suffering hallucinations. He was admitted to Baylor where doctors there quickly diagnosed him with acute liver failure. On October 2, he deteriorated further, and had a breathing tube threaded down his throat. He was on a ventilator to breathe, and medications to support his blood pressure.

His condition was critical. Pennington was at the top of the liver transplant list, but Levy doubted he could stay alive long enough to get an offer, much less to survive the risky liver transplant. He set up a meeting with Charlotte Pennington, Robert's grandmother, which occurred by Robert's bedside in the ICU in the middle of the night. Charlotte recalled being frightened. She had been praying for her grandchild, praying that he could hold on long enough to get a liver. Now this big transplant surgeon with the slicked black hair was telling her that his only chance might be provided by a pig. Charlotte still has her blue spiral notebook where she wrote down some of the words Levy spoke: "Uncharted territory. Not done at Baylor before." Nevertheless, Levy thought it was Robert's best chance. After a sleepless night, Charlotte agreed.

The next day, a fifteen-week-old, 118-pound transgenic pig was brought to the OR in the animal lab. Levy removed the liver, just like he hoped to do to Robert in the near future. He brought the beautiful, glistening brown organ to Robert's bedside, and at 4:10 p.m. hooked up the catheters that would divert the blood from Robert's circulatory system into the pig liver, and then out of the pig liver back into Robert. The clamps were removed, and the liver pinked up immediately. The blood flowed through it at two liters per minute. Robert's condition seemed to stabilize. A few hours after starting the perfusion, Robert received an offer for a human liver from nearby Houston. He received just under seven hours of pig-liver perfusion before he was ultimately disconnected and prepared for the human transplant. His surgery went without a hitch, and two years later Robert was as healthy as ever. Robert and Charlotte are convinced that the pig saved his life. Charlotte keeps a snapshot of it in her scrapbook. It was given to her by one of the animal handlers. Although Nextran doesn't name their pigs, the Baylor animal care team had named it Sweetie Pie. Charlotte refers to Sweetie Pie as "the pig that was sacrificed to save Robert."[14]

* * * * *

Less than three hours up I-95 (and I-287) from Nextran, a group of Yale scientists started their own biotechnology company that they named Alexion Pharmaceuticals. Their strategy was similar to White's, but to distinguish themselves they settled on injecting the genes for two complement regulatory proteins and one enzyme to decrease the expression of Alpha Gal. By 1995, Alexion was performing tests with both perfusion of human organs *ex-vivo* and transplantation of hearts and kidneys into baboons. Although their results were similar to Nextran's and not as impressive as Imutran's, all three groups successfully prevented hyperacute rejection in their models. Alexion was formed nine years after Imutran, but was the first to receive patent protection in the United States (Imutran had already received patent protection for its pigs in Europe, and filings in the United States were pending). Alexion garnered interest from its own major investor, United States Surgical. In 1995, the large surgical equipment manufacturer made a 9.5 percent equity investment in Alexion, and in return gained exclusive manufacturing, marketing, and sales rights to the genetically engineered pigs.

* * * * *

Money was pouring in to these companies, to the tune of hundreds of millions of dollars. White told one newspaper that he expected trials in humans to begin within two years. It seemed like nothing could hold them back, according to the interviews and articles in the press, and the actions of the deep-pocketed biotech companies. And yet, the outcomes in animal experiments—the actual data—told a different story. Transplant survival in these preclinical models was still measured in weeks to months. As ground-breaking as it was to create genetically modified animals, it was starting to feel unlikely that simply focusing on complement regulation in the pigs would be enough to sustain a xenotransplantation long term. Novel and efficacious strategies would need to be developed.

* * * * *

One of the biggest draws for David Sachs to return to Boston in 1991 was the opportunity to finally move his xenotransplantation experiments into large animals—using his own herd of mini-swine as donors and monkeys as recipients. Ever since he had started breeding the mini-swine, Sachs wanted to start using them as donors for xeno experiments. But he knew that these experiments were just too expensive to fund with NIH grants. His move to Boston would finally give him an opportunity. Some of his support would come from his large financial startup package that brought him to Massachusetts General Hospital. But even more important, when he arrived in Boston, he began a collaboration with Biotransplant, a biotech startup focused on solving the shortage of organs for transplant. Sachs would be their primary scientific collaborator. In one of Sachs's first meetings with CEO Elliot Lebowitz, Sachs sounded a note of caution, warning how expensive these xeno experiments were going to be. Lebowitz didn't bat an eye. He knew what he had with Sachs, his unique herd of mini-swine, and the incredible science that Sachs and his collaborators had been producing. "That's what we're here for," Lebowitz said. "We want to get this moving."[15]

Sachs now proceeded with a multipronged approach to his translational research program. His labs occupied the massive ninth floor of the Charlestown Navy Yard, sitting on the inner harbor with a view of the Boston skyline. The lab included extensive space for investigators and technicians, benches for performing experiments, and two fully stocked operating rooms that ran more efficiently than many human ORs. There was housing for numerous primates and mini-swine just down the hall from the ORs.

Four floors down, on the fifth floor, sat Megan Sykes's outfit, with a similar blueprint to Sachs's, only the type of animals used for experimentation differed. The animal rooms in the Sykes lab were filled with cage upon cage of mice and rats. Sykes, an absolute genius, would conduct tolerance and xenotransplant experiments on the rodents, using skin grafts, cell transplants, and even heart and kidney transplants sewn under the microscope. The xeno experiments in Sykes's lab primarily involved mice and rats, but she also took advantage of Sachs's inbred herd of mini-swine, transplanting pig skin or cells onto/into the rodents. Each time Sykes's lab developed new protocols that worked, Sachs's group would try to perfect them in pig or primate allotransplants, or—if the results were particularly promising—in pig-to-primate xenotransplants.

As Sachs and Sykes were uncovering the mechanisms behind the tolerance protocols, they kept coming back to the role of the thymus, the organ that serves to educate the T cells, the central component of the immune response. It occurred to these brilliant scientists that maybe they could harness the thymus in a different way. Could it be possible to transplant the thymus from a donor to a recipient? There would be a few advantages to such a protocol. First, it might remove the need for radiation to the recipient, a component of the conditioning protocols that seemed to be required for success. Sachs knew that radiation was not a popular treatment for patients, and was anxious to find a protocol that didn't utilize it. Perhaps if the thymus itself was transplanted along with a transplanted organ, and the recipient underwent T cell depletion and removal of the native thymus at the same operation, the transplanted thymus might become the center for continuing education and delete any maturing immune cells that would react against the donor and the recipient. It was worth a try.

The thymus transplant project benefited from the arrival of Kazuhiko (Kaz) Yamada, a brilliant urologist and scientist trained in Japan who was performing a research fellowship before returning to Japan. Yamada is an uber confident researcher who is driven to solve scientific puzzles with near obsession. He always knows what experiment he wants to do next and does not let barriers stand in his way. He is as confident in his surgical ability as he is in his scientific knowledge.

Yamada and Sachs embarked on a mission to figure out the best way to transplant a thymus with a kidney. They performed multiple iterations, transplanting lobes of this beefy gland into various locations in the recipient (under the skin, into the abdominal fat termed the "omentum," under the kidney capsule of the recipient, into the neck of the recipient). Every time they did it, when they would return a few weeks later to examine the gland it would be replaced by fibrous tissue and inflammatory cells of the host.

They came up with two solutions to the problem. The first was to give the gland time to vascularize prior to the actual transplant. Yamada brought a potential donor pig to the operating room weeks prior to a planned transplant, removed a lobe of the thymus gland, opened its belly, and inserted the gland under the capsule of the animal's own kidney. The pig then recovered from anesthesia and resumed its normal activities. Six weeks later Yamada returned to the OR and removed the new organ, now termed a "thymokidney," and examined it under a microscope. He found the gland was healthy with a normal architecture and functioning thymocytes. Further experiments confirmed that not only was the thymus alive, but it was functioning as well, educating immature T cells as if nothing had happened.

Next, Yamada created a few more thymokidneys in fresh pigs, allowing the new organ to mature for six weeks or more. He then transplanted the organs across various pre-determined MHC mismatches into recipient mini-swine, removing the recipient thymus and depleting the circulating T cells with antibodies. The transplants themselves were technically like any other kidney transplant, with the artery and vein of the kidney sewn into the artery and vein in the abdomen of the recipient. The kidneys functioned right away, and over time, they showed that the new thymus was working, helping to prevent graft rejection. Yamada spent the next few years trying to make this protocol work across more stringent MHC mismatches in pigs, and then eventually transferring the protocol into primates.[16]

While Yamada focused much of his energy on this set of projects, and Sykes continued to explore the mechanisms of tolerance and xenotransplantation in small animal models, Sachs and his team began their xenotransplant experiments in the pig-to-monkey model in earnest. They tried everything they could think of in those first few years. Their research focused on strategies to reduce the amount of Alpha Gal antibody prior to transplant, after transplant, or both. They targeted complement, first with CVF and then with transgenic pigs from David White. They tried all available immunosuppression. They tried bone marrow transplants, thymectomies, and thymus transplants. They used radiation, splenectomies, and even spleen transplants. None of it worked. No matter what they did, the natural antibodies would come back and lead to destruction of the transplanted organ. They used various versions of plasmapheresis where recipient monkeys and baboons had their blood filtered and all of the antibodies removed before, during, and after a transplant, but it just did not work.

By the mid-1990s, Sachs had a discussion with David Cooper, and convinced him to come join him in Boston. Cooper had grown tired of running a clinical transplant center by this point and wanted to focus his energy on making xenotransplantation a reality. Despite all the failures, Cooper believed it was going to succeed, and wanted to be part of the team that made it happen. Sachs, always the optimist, felt the same way. Cooper took a spot in Sachs's lab, running the section on heart xenotransplantation using the mini-swine, while Yamada continued with the efforts with kidney transplantation.

Sachs knew by now that no matter what treatment he employed on the recipient side, it would never be enough to prevent destruction of the transplant by preformed antibody. He also knew that David White's transgenic pigs, derived from Astrid, also weren't going to do the trick. If pigs were ever going to be the donors for humans, he would have to find a way to get rid of Alpha Gal. But could it be done?

* * * * *

In the early 1990s, it was not possible to generate a large animal with a particular gene knocked out. Some basic gene-targeting technology did exist that would allow injection of a simple strand of DNA into a nucleus with a small chance it would disrupt a gene already present. But a scientist might start with millions of cells and only succeed in knocking out a specific gene of interest in one cell! That might sound like the most tedious and painstaking job ever, but some persistent scientists and technicians were able to succeed. The problem was, once you had the cell, what could you do with it?

In 1981, researchers working in Switzerland published the first report of a cloned mouse.[17] They harvested undifferentiated stem cells from a fertilized mouse embryo. The nuclei of these embryonic stem cells could then be injected into fertilized egg cells from different mice, after the nuclear material was sucked out of these egg cells. These fertilized eggs would then divide in culture becoming embryos, which could be implanted into the uteri of surrogate mice. This process, termed "nuclear transfer," or cloning, was burdensome but occasionally successful. Over time the process became more efficient, and it was possible to utilize unfertilized eggs to generate a clone. Given how inexpensive and available mice are, how short their gestation is (twenty days), and how large a litter can be (up to twelve pups), cloning mice became practical.

In 1984, Steen Willadsen, a Dutch researcher working at Cambridge in England took cells from lamb embryos and used electricity to fuse them with sheep egg cells that had their nuclei removed. He placed these new cells in culture and they began dividing, and he implanted them into the uterus of a sheep. This sheep gave birth to three live lambs. These were the first successfully cloned large animals.[18] That was a major step forward in cloning, but he was unable to identify stem cells from the lamb embryos that would grow in culture until they were fused with the sheep eggs, which meant he couldn't perform any genetic modifications on these cloned animals. In 1987, a team that included the scientist Randal Prather in Missouri succeeded in cloning two calves (named Fusion and Copy), using the same techniques as Willadsen.[19]

1996 was a landmark year in the history of cloning. Ian Wilmut and Keith Campbell, researchers working at the Roslin Institute outside of Edinburgh and associated with the University of Edinburgh, had two major breakthroughs. In the first, they successfully cultured embryonic sheep cells in the lab, getting them to divide and grow. They then were able to take the nuclei from these cultured stem cells and transfer them into enucleated sheep egg cells, and implant these new embryos into surrogate sheep. Two lambs were born, named Megan and Morag. This raised the possibility that knockout large animals could eventually be generated.[20] On the technical side, these cultured embryonic cells were fickle and difficult to keep dividing in culture, so the likelihood of successful gene editing with the rudimentary techniques available at that time was a long shot.

Later this same year, the Roslin researchers accomplished something even bigger—they removed the nucleus from the mammary gland of a six-year-old ewe (female sheep) and transferred it into an enucleated sheep egg. After cell division, embryos were implanted into a surrogate sheep and a cloned sheep was born.[21] This remarkable sheep was named Dolly. (As it was derived from mammary gland cells, the Edinburgh team chose the name to honor Dolly Parton.) The experiment required all the persistence any good geneticist needed—the success followed 276 failures. Never before had an adult somatic cell (differentiated, non-reproductive cell) been used to clone another living creature. It proved that differentiated cells can in fact return to their embryonic state and turn on genes that had been silenced as the cell differentiated into its final cell-type. It had previously been assumed that only stem cells could accomplish this feat, which had limited the potential for cloning.

The Roslin team didn't stop there. They inserted the DNA-encoding human Factor IX, a gene that encodes a clotting factor deficient in Hemophilia B, into sheep skin cells growing in culture. Once they confirmed that they had sheep skin cells generating human Factor IX, they performed nuclear transfer of these transgenic cells into a sheep egg and placed the embryo in a surrogate. In 1997, Polly, the first transgenic large animal made by genetic modification of a somatic cell and nuclear transfer was born. She made human Factor IX in her milk.[22] The era of generating transgenic large animals with cloning had begun.

* * * * *

The Roslin Institute supported scientists that were academics at heart, and they all had appointments as professors at the University of Edinburgh. They wanted their findings to improve human health, but were not the type to leave the lab to commercialize their intellectual property. In 1987, PPL Therapeutics was formed to help accomplish that, with a focus on making therapeutic human proteins generated in transgenic animals. The company went public in 1996, timed with the publication of Dolly, immediately recognized as one of the biggest scientific advancements in the last century. PPL Therapeutics was further bolstered by the birth of Polly one year later. The commercialization potential of their transgenic technology was obvious, and money poured in from every imaginable source. They opened subsidiaries all around the world, including large pig farms across the United Kingdom, Europe and New Zealand, and one in the small rural town of Blacksburg, Virginia.

While xenotransplantation was not on the mind of Ian Wilmut and his team when they cloned Dolly, the leadership of PPL did immediately grasp the potential. Executives at PPL realized that they were just a few years from being able to knockout Alpha Gal and add any number of more complex genetic modifications to a cloned pig. The potential six-billion-dollar yearly market valuation was enticing to the PPL C-Suite. The Edinburgh researchers already had their hands full, so it made sense to identify a different location for this novel work. The Blacksburg group was already working on cloning a cow, a project they had started a few years before. How hard would it be to clone a pig on the side?

* * * * *

David Ayares had never intended to spend his life working in xenotransplantation (although he should have, given his name was David). He grew up in the Midwest, where his dad sold insurance, and his mother stayed home to raise him, his brother, and his sister. When he was young, Ayares thought he might like to be a veterinarian, but then in middle school he had a science class with Mr. Manny, who brought the field to life for him. From that day he knew he wanted to be a scientist. As a freshman in high school, he was already taking science classes with the seniors, and the teachers didn't know what to do with him. He matriculated at Purdue University, where he majored in microbiology.

It was there, in the lab studying bacteria and yeast, that he had his first exposure to the biologic phenomena of homologous recombination.[23] This is a process where genetic information can be exchanged between two similar strands of DNA. It happens in cells naturally, as a technique to repair abnormal and accidental breaks in DNA. It is the same process that bacteria utilize to transfer genes for antibiotic resistance between strains. It also occurs when organisms (including humans) are making sperm or egg cells, allowing genetic variation in offspring. After fertilization of an egg, paired DNA material from the male and female parents align, and similar DNA sequences can cross over from one chromosome to the other. This subtle "shuffling of genetic materials, just like some gentle shuffling of a deck of cards" is an important way that genetic variation is introduced in populations.[24] This concept had been recognized for many years, although the exact details of recombination were still being worked out in the early 1980s.

After graduating from Purdue in 1982, Ayares pursued a PhD in mammalian genetics at the University of Illinois Medical Center, which he completed in 1987. This degree coincided with the seminal discovery by Oliver Smithies of how to use homologous recombination to modify the mouse genome.[25] Smithies demonstrated that he could create a DNA fragment (or gene) that was similar to the portion of the gene he wanted to edit. He would inject the DNA fragment into the nucleus of the cell, where it may recombine with the cell's DNA and replace the original gene with the injected DNA fragment. The technique was inefficient and inaccurate, with the potential for off-target effects. The probability of the injected fragment landing in the intended spot was on the order of one in a million. But unlike the technique White had used for his hDAF pigs, it could be used to knock out a gene and replace it with a nonfunctional fragment of DNA. Given the inefficiency, it could not be performed in fertilized eggs, the same eggs White used to inject his hDAF gene. But in somatic cells that are dividing in culture, with a tenacious scientist, it would be possible to knock a gene out.

Ayares spent his PhD years mastering these techniques, continuing his training in a postdoctoral fellowship at the Massachusetts Institute of Technology in Boston. He was finally ready to get a job at the tender age of thirty. By then he had a wife and two children, and it was time to make some money. He decided to go into industry rather than academia, with a plan to use gene therapy to study mouse models of human disease. He started at the transgenic mouse facility at Abbott Labs in Chicago, using homologous recombination to knock out genes that might be important in known human diseases. The goal was to find therapeutic targets, but his bosses at Abbott were never sure what to do with the mice. After a few aimless years at Abbott, Ayares moved down the road to Baxter Health Care, where they were performing gene therapy on pig islet cells to identify a treatment for diabetes. After two years, Ayares saw that Baxter was losing interest in gene therapy, and he was losing interest in working for them. One morning in 1996, he was sitting in the cafeteria, sipping his coffee and flipping through the classified ads in a scientific journal, wondering how he was going to fill his day, and more importantly how he was going to continue supporting his family. He noticed one job posting that looked interesting. Some Scottish company was looking for a scientist with experience in homologous recombination. PPL Therapeutics. He had no idea what they made, or what they wanted to edit, but he had heard Edinburgh was nice. Next thing he knew he was on a plane to Scotland.

At his interview in PPL headquarters, Ayares was told that their company was primarily focused on generating human therapeutic proteins in the milk of transgenic animals. They had acquired a facility in Blacksburg, Virginia to work on cows. They were working with sheep on the island, given the mad cow disease epidemic in the United Kingdom, but thought there might be some important protein targets that would work better in cows. The challenge was that large animals had not yet been cloned from anything but embryonic cells, cells that Ayares knew he couldn't genetically modify. But the executives at PPL didn't seem worried. They were confident the science was moving quickly, and before long these problems would be solved. Ayares wasn't convinced, but he was ready for something new and figured Virginia would be a nice place to raise his family. With Virginia Tech nearby, there would be other jobs there if this one didn't work out.

Ayares took his family on a one-week vacation in February of 1996, before starting his job at PPL. He fittingly was reading *Jurassic Park* by Michael Crichton, in which scientists used genetic engineering to recreate extinct dinosaurs. He remembers laughing to himself, knowing it would be impossible to clone an animal from just a little bit of DNA. Then, in the *New York Times*, slapped across the front page, was the headline from an article by Gina Kolata: "Scientist Reports First Cloning Ever Of Adult Mammal."[26] "In a feat that may be the one bit of genetic engineering that has been anticipated and dreaded more than any other, researchers in Britain are reporting that they have cloned an adult mammal for the first time. The group, led by Dr. Ian Wilmut, a 52-year-old embryologist at the Roslin Institute in Edinburgh, created a lamb using DNA from an adult sheep. The achievement shocked leading researchers who had said it could not be done." Much of the rest of the article focused on the impact this might have on animal husbandry, noting that if cows could be cloned, it might be possible to genetically engineer cows that would be milk super-producers. Then the article veered into the macabre, discussing the potential to clone humans including the dead. Ayares looked over at his half-read copy of *Jurassic Park* and wondered if he should bother finishing it. It suddenly seemed so banal. Now he couldn't wait to get to work. It was time to make a super-producer milk cow.

* * * * *

"'An end to the chronic organ shortage is now in sight,' PPL's managing director, Mr. Ron James, said yesterday, adding that 'all the known technical hurdles have now been overcome.'" This quote was from a press release shared with major news networks on March 15, 2000.[27] The announcement marked the first time a pig was cloned from an adult somatic cell. The project took a bit longer than PPL anticipated; they stuck with their plan of cloning cows in Blacksburg, which was ultimately successful. Then they moved on to pigs, having convinced their board and investors that the $6 billion xenotransplant market was in reach. While Ayares spent his time learning pig genetics and gene editing via homologous recombination in adult pig cells, other scientists in the lab attempted to clone a pig.

It presented some unexpected challenges due to physiological differences between cows and sheep, but over time success was achieved. After many iterations, the Blacksburg subsidiary produced Millie (for the new millennium), Christa (after Christian Barnard), Alexis and Carrel (after Alexis Carrel, the brilliant scientist who performed the first vascular anastomosis and many transplants in animals at the turn of the twentieth century;), and

Dotcom (because "any association with dot-coms right now seems to have a very positive influence on a company's valuation," Ron James said). James stated that they were looking to raise $20 million to reach clinical trials within four years. PPL further announced that Ayares had knocked out the gene for Alpha Gal in pig cells, so the generation of Alpha Gal knockout pigs was right around the corner.

The announcement was not accompanied by a peer-reviewed paper submitted to any scientific journal—PPL had no interest in sharing its proprietary techniques with anyone in the scientific community. They knew they weren't the only ones trying to generate a knockout pig, and were aware that one particular company was most likely just as far along as they were. That knowledge was the impetus for the next line in their press release. "We are unaware of any other group that has as comprehensive an approach to xenotransplantation as PPL," said James. "All the known technical hurdles have been overcome. It is now a case of combining the various strategies into one male and one female pig, and breeding from these."

The goal of the press release was to raise money. Ayares, who was now the vice president of research and development at PPL was forthright about this, sharing that they were in discussion with drug companies, venture capitalists, and investment bankers. He also revealed his plans to publish the details of pig cloning in a major scientific journal, either *Science* or *Nature*. Ayares commented that the process of cloning pigs was more challenging than expected, and it took several hundred attempts. What he didn't share was that they had to perform nuclear transfer twice, first transferring the contents of an adult cell into an enucleated egg, and then a second transfer into a fertilized egg that had also been enucleated. They wouldn't disclose this detail for another six months.

* * * * *

One person who read the press release carefully was David Sachs. He believed in sharing his data and techniques with everyone in the field and found this strategy distasteful. He wasn't naïve and knew the importance of protecting his discoveries, but he would never go to the press before publishing in the scientific literature. Sachs wasn't running a biotech company; he was running a lab. The first call he made after reading the release was Elliot Lebowitz, the CEO of BioTransplant. "Elliot, whatever it costs, you've got to get that technology."[28] It probably would have cost $20 million, maybe more. But fortunately for Sachs, that wouldn't be necessary. BioTransplant had formed a collaboration with Randall Prather, the co-director of the National Swine Research and Resource Center at the University of Missouri's College of Agriculture, Food, and Natural Resources, and himself a giant in the field of livestock cloning. Sachs could hardly believe his ears when Prather told him that he, too, had cloned a pig. No cute name, no fancy announcement, but they had done it.

Sachs knew something else, a piece of information he was sitting on since 1998. He knew that Robert Hawley, the principal scientist at BioTransplant, had been using homologous recombination to target the Alpha Gal gene in an adult somatic cell taken from Sachs's mini-swine pigs. His goal was to replace the gene with inactive DNA. When he started the project, he was told he had a one-in-ten-million chance to succeed. After six years, countless attempts, and a near maniacal obsession with the task, he succeeded. This was two years before PPL announced their cloned pigs. He had knocked out the Alpha Gal gene in one of the two copies expressed in the chromosomes of the cell (with a copy coming from the mother and the father). Hawley had been sitting on these cells for two years, with nothing to do with them. They all had understood that when Dolly was generated in 1996, a pig couldn't be far behind, and when that happened, they would be ready to run.

The next year at Sachs's Transplantation Biology Research Center at Massachusetts General Hospital was filled with anticipation and stress for him and his team. They continued their experiments on tolerance using chimerism and continued to develop novel ways to induce tolerance with thymus transplant. In addition to the composite thymokidney, Yamada began transplanting the thymus as an isolated vascular organ. This challenging operation required removing the thymus from the donor while preserving its blood supply from the internal carotid artery and internal jugular vein. He then would remove the thymus from the recipient and anastomose the new thymus into either the neck (sewing the vessels to the recipient carotid artery and internal jugular vein) or the abdomen (sewing the vessels onto the aorta and inferior vena cava) of the recipient. The new thymus transplants functioned just like the composite thymokidney.[29] These thymus transplants would be relevant for the xenotransplant of organs like the heart, lungs, liver, and pancreas, where a composite organ wasn't possible.

Nearly every day, Sachs would wait for updates from Missouri and BioTransplant. He knew that Prather was trying to clone pigs using the knockout cells missing a copy of the Alpha Gal gene. He also knew that Hawley was painstakingly trying to knock out the other copy of the Alpha Gal gene from the pig cells. If he failed, Prather would have to mate the single knockout pigs together, eventually leading to homozygous knockouts by breeding. Every morning, Sachs nervously opened the newspaper waiting to read a press release announcing that Ayares and his team had succeeded with a knockout.

In September of 2001, Prather reported that a litter was born with single Alpha Gal knockouts. A second successful litter followed in October, giving him male and female knockouts. Once the pigs became of age, Prather began breeding them together. As long as they bred well, standard Mendelian genetics would predict that one in four progeny would be homozygous knockouts for the Alpha Gal gene, or complete knockouts. It was just a matter of time. Prather, Hawley, and the team at BioTransplant put their work together and submitted it for publication to *Science*, the premier scientific journal in the world. They weren't going to play the public relations game that so annoyed them when PPL did it.

As Sachs's team waited for their groundbreaking *Science* publication to come out, slated for an online release on January 3, 2002,[30] PPL knew it had to act. "The promise of xenotransplantation is now a reality."[31] So said Alan Colman, PPL's head of research. In a virtual tribute to White, Ayares told the press the Alpha Gal heterozygous knockout pigs were born on Christmas Day, and christened the litter Noel, Angel, Star, Joy, and Mary. Ayares went on: "This advance provides a near term solution for overcoming the shortage of human organs for transplants as well as insulin-producing cells to cure diabetes." Ayares did include one additional tidbit in interviews with the press. He mentioned that PPL was looking to spin off its US-Blacksburg division and was seeking a buyer. That was news to Sachs and his team at

BioTransplant. Why was PPL looking to spin off its xeno division, when it was so close to having the Alpha Gal knockout on the ground?

Both groups had single knockout clones and were madly trying to breed them together to yield homozygous knockouts. In Sachs's mind, he had an advantage—his clones were on the mini-swine background, with organs more appropriate for humans. He also could control the MHC of these animals, which he predicted would prove important in defining immunosuppression strategies and even tolerance in the future. But in the end, all that mattered was getting the full knockouts. Hawley wasn't one to sit and wait for the breeding to happen, for nature to take its course. He used homologous recombination on literally millions of single knockout cells and was never able to knock out the other Alpha Gal gene. He searched for a different strategy. He harvested cells from the single knockout pigs and grew them out in the lab. After analyzing millions of those cells that were growing in culture, he was able to identify a small number that had spontaneously mutated and lost the other copy of the gene! He sent those off to Prather.

On August 22, 2002, PPL circulated another press release.[32] The world's first double-knockout piglets, expressing no Alpha Gal, were on the ground. Four pigs had been born on July 25, 2002. "'The next step in the ongoing research will be conducted in collaboration with the University of Pittsburgh's Thomas E. Starzl Transplantation Institute. Organs and cells from these double-knockout pigs will be used in pivotal transplantation studies aimed at testing for elimination of hyperacute rejection and long term survival of these xenografts,' the company said." PPL was working with Starzl! That was news to Sachs. Starzl was a legend by this time, and was the most aggressive innovator the world of transplant had ever known.

On November 18, Prather announced to the team at BioTransplant that it had succeeded. The first double knockout from their group was now on the ground. Though this wasn't their practice previously, they decided to name this pig. After much discussion, they settled on Goldie. More knockout pigs followed shortly thereafter. The Boston group was now in business, and the team couldn't wait to start transplant experiments. They had to sit on their hands while Goldie and the other knockouts grew old enough (and big enough) to be ready for use. They could only imagine what was going on in Virginia (and Pittsburgh).

This moment in time, at the end of 2002 and the beginning of 2003, should have been the most exhilarating in the lives of these two Davids—Sachs and Ayares. It certainly was exciting. But unexpectedly, it was also the most stressful, the most perilous in their journey to make xenotransplantation a reality. Just at the point where real breakthroughs seemed imminent, the door to xenotransplantation was rapidly closing. Dark, cold winds were blowing through the xenotransplant world, bringing stress and uncertainty to Boston and Virginia.

5 UNCERTAIN PERIL (1995–2004)

Even during the most exciting moments of the race for the xeno in the 1990s, there were always dark undercurrents that had the potential to become existential threats to the very discipline itself. The first was the animal rights movement that was becoming more aggressive with every press release predicting that trials were imminent. The second was the pace at which the science was advancing. Could milestones come quickly enough to keep the attention (and the money) of the large companies that were funding the efforts, looking for profits rather than scientific publications? The third was the threat of infection. Transplanting animal organs into humans had the potential to unleash a novel virus or bacteria never seen before in humans that would have the capacity to evade the human immune system. The risk of a deadly pandemic always seemed unlikely to xeno researchers, who were quick to point out that humans had lived in close contact with pigs and other farm animals for thousands of years. Each one of these risks seemed manageable on its own, but if they all reached a crescendo at the same time, would xenotransplantation survive?

"The relationship of Homo sapiens (humans) to the other animals is one of unremitting exploitation. We employ their work; we eat and wear them. We exploit them to serve our superstitions: whereas we used to sacrifice them to our gods and tear out their entrails in order to foresee the future, we now sacrifice them to science, and experiment on their entrails in the hope—or on the mere off chance—that we might thereby see a little more clearly into the present."—Brigid Brophy, *Sunday Times*, October 1965.[1]

When these powerful words appeared in the newspaper of record in the United Kingdom in 1965, they reached a sympathetic audience. Supporters of animal rights have a long history in the UK, dating as far back as 1875, when the first anti-vivisection organization was founded. Shortly thereafter, in 1898, a second group emerged—the British Union for Abolition of Vivisection. This organization remains active to this day, has grown in size and public support, and has had many political successes that have led to more stringent rules governing the use of animals in research in the UK.

Its stance on the use of animals in medical experimentation is that it is morally unjustifiable. "To inflict suffering on defenceless animals during experiments is wrong. We do not have the right to experiment on or use animals for our benefit." The group has sponsored peaceful protests against the use of animals in science over the years, and has successfully raised awareness about the rights of animals, a concept that was not even considered throughout most of the developed world in the 1900s.

The animal rights movement continued to grow throughout the 1900s, perhaps best personified by the Oxford Vegetarians, a group of philosophy students who published their treatise in the topic in 1971, under the title "Animals, Men and Morals."[2] While this publication had a rather limited effect on British society, it did inspire one of its younger members, Peter Singer, to publish a review of the work, followed by his seminal book *Animal Liberation* in 1975.[3] To this day this is considered the bible of the animal rights movement. It was in this book that Singer popularized the term "speciesism," "the belief that we are entitled to treat members of other species in a way in which it would be wrong to treat members of our own species," a term that had been coined by one of the original members of the Oxford Vegetarians. The comparisons to racism were obvious, and were also explicitly delineated in the book.

* * * * *

It was in this environment that Imutran pushed ahead with its pig-to-primate experiments. The majority of its experimental transplant surgeries were conducted at Huntington Life Sciences, a contract research organization with a facility located nearby. Numerous animal rights groups focused their energy and efforts at exposing the work conducted at this facility and across the United Kingdom, with daily raucous demonstrations and attempts to infiltrate the labs themselves.

White was the target of animal rights attacks for most of his career, ever since his work on cyclosporine in the late 1970s and early 1980s. Those attacks, however, intensified in the 1990s in response to his xenotransplantation work and his many appearances on radio shows, television programs, and in newspapers. His untethered optimism and predictions for the future worked against him with this audience. The concept of xenotransplantation captured the imagination of animal rights activists, and not a in a good way. The very idea of breeding animals to supply organs for humans reeked of speciesism. The notion of genetically modifying these animals added to the dystopian nature of the imagined horror.

"The potential harm of genetic modification is of a different magnitude from the changes which occur in normal breeding. Regular breeding produces tiny changes over generations, whereas genetic modification is immediate, with potentially lots of consequences for the animal. In addition, in genetic research of the type being carried out here, genes are swapped between species of animals. That is not natural."[4]

White was the public face of xenotransplantation in the UK (and worldwide), which put him in the sights of animal activists. He often had police protection and would even wear bulletproof vests at public appearances. His house was vandalized multiple times, including one particular incident occurring when he was abroad. His house was flooded and sustained thousands of dollars of damage, with loss of many irreplaceable heirlooms. Offensive and hostile statements were scrawled on his walls threatening him and his family.

Imutran's "levee" broke in September of 2000, when the "Diaries of Despair" was published first online by the animal rights group "Uncaged Campaign," and then picked up by every major UK newspaper.[5] Confidential reports, communications, letters, and animal study reports were leaked from inside Imutran to Uncaged Campaign. Over 1,200 pages of documents were disclosed in all, and they left an ugly impression of the research being conducted at Imutran.

The report described graphic experimentation on numerous animals, and highlighted the government's role in approving these studies. *The Guardian*, a leading newspaper in the UK, summarized a portion of it as follows:

> To the dismay of animal rights activists, the documents reveal how primates were used in the search for a solution to the chronic global shortage of human organs for transplant. Baboons were transported from the African savannahs to die in steel cages the size of toilet cubicles. The documents show that a quarter of the primates died from "technical failures."
>
> Researchers describe how monkeys and baboons died in fits of vomiting and diarrhoea. Symptoms included violent spasms, bloody discharges, grinding teeth and uncontrollable, manic eye movements. Other animals retreated within themselves, lying still in their cages until put of their misery.[6]

Although White and others at Imutran remained discreet after these documents hit the press, he had been the staunchest of defenders for animal research beforehand. "As far as the animal rights activists are concerned, I accept that they have a right to reject animal experimentation. I accept they have a right to reject for themselves the product of medical research on animals. But I don't accept that they have a right to prevent the population at large from benefiting from what that research can bring. And even an animal rights activist, when he's sick, goes to the doctor and says 'help me.' If the animal rights people had their way, they would stop all progress in medical research. There is not a single medical advance that's currently being placed in hospitals that hasn't gone through animal research. You stop animal research, you stop medical advance, it's as simple as that. I find that an unacceptable position for anybody to take up."[7]

As much as White tried to control the backlash, he couldn't compete with the images that were generated, both by words and photos, in the bombshell report. Perhaps the largest nail in the coffin was that in the end, the xenotransplant outcomes in the primates just weren't very good. "In five years of experiments, causing severe suffering to hundreds of primates and sacrificing thousands of pigs, Imutran and Novartis managed to squeeze average survival times up by a couple of weeks. Very little progress was made in overcoming the profound immunological obstacles to xenotransplantation. Is the notion of functioning pig organ transplants nothing more than scientific arrogance driven by personal ambition and commercial greed? Transforming organs from pigs into human organs appears to be nothing more than a modern form of alchemy."[8]

White was frustrated with his portrayal in the press, threats to his family's safety, and the onerous regulations that the British government had already placed on conducting animal research even before the leak of these documents—regulations that were far stricter than those in most other countries, certainly more than in the United States. Novartis agreed. Just one month after publication of "Diaries of Despair," Novartis decided to pull its backing of Imutran and move its funding across the pond to David Sachs's group in Boston. They proceeded to buy two-thirds of BioTransplant with a multimillion-dollar investment, changing the name of the company to "Immerge BioTherapeutics." Novartis promised Immerge ten million dollars per year for three years, with the hope that by the end of that period, human trials would at least be in sight.

Most other pharmaceutical and medical device companies came to a similar conclusion, and either pulled their facilities from the UK or decided not to invest in research there. They publicly claimed that this move had nothing to do with the protests and negativity in the press, and had more to do with the slow progress in making xenotransplantation work. It was becoming clear to the scientists at Novartis that simply regulating complement was not going to blow open the multibillion-dollar field of xenotransplantation in just a couple of years. White decided to leave the UK and was recruited to London, Ontario as a professor of xenotransplantation at Western University. His research would continue but his time in the spotlight had ended.

* * * * *

When Novartis shifted its financial commitment to BioTransplant (now Immerge) and proudly announced the three-year investment pledge, whispers of pulling the plug on xeno entirely were audible well outside of the Swiss conference rooms where Novartis executives convened. Outcomes in the animal experiments just hadn't achieved the results the company was expecting when it purchased Imutran five years earlier. Sachs knew time was limited—he spent his days pushing the research as fast as it would go, and his nights endlessly writing grants and scrounging for money to fund his large and preposterously expensive lab.

Circumstances were just as tenuous for David Ayares in Blacksburg. He had joined the Virginia subsidiary of PPL in 1996, just on the heels of the cloning of Dolly. By the time the first pigs were cloned in 2000, he was an executive vice president and head of research, essentially running the show in Virginia. Unlike Sachs, Ayares was a geneticist and now an expert in cloning. When the first cloned pigs hit the ground in 2000, followed by PPL's massive press release, Ayares was surprised to see this was the number one story in the world. Film crews from all over the world converged on this small rural town in Virginia to get a shot of these clones that would eventually save us all. One of the first calls Ayares received was from Thomas Starzl himself. Now retired from the practice of clinical medicine but devoting all of his prodigious resources and inexhaustible energy to research, Starzl told Ayares the path to clinical xenotransplantation was now possible, and he wanted to collaborate. He was confident the Alpha Gal knockout would blow the hatches on xeno. If there was anyone that had the gravitas to take on a risky and ethically provocative endeavor like xeno—the drive to push it through the regulatory, economic, and social barriers and the access to potential patients—it was Starzl.

Despite all of that, Ayares was spending increasing quantities of his time fighting for dollars rather than editing pig cells and cloning pigs. How could that be? There were a number of factors. There were the animal rights protestors. There was the inability to obtain long-term survival in primates, although the promise of a quantum improvement seemed just around the corner. But now, a new and stronger headwind was blowing in the face of the xeno researchers, and it was known by the unfortunate acronym "PERV": Porcine Endogenous Retroviruses.

* * * * *

The risk of transmitting an animal virus into humans has always been a concern with xenotransplantation. Animals were long known to carry various infections novel to humans, and periodically a pathogen would jump across this species barrier and lead to a deadly pandemic. The one that has raised the most fear in the modern era is HIV, which originated in chimpanzees and was near-universally fatal until the late 1990s. Pigs were known to harbor certain unique viruses, including porcine cytomegalovirus and versions of a herpesvirus not seen in humans. At the same time, they were considered "cleaner" than primates. They do not carry HIV or primate Herpes B virus, both devastating in humans. Pigs and humans have interacted closely for ten thousand years. Over that period, few infectious diseases have jumped from pigs to humans. Any herd of pigs as organ donors would be bred in the cleanest of conditions, with physical assessment and testing for viruses frequently. This seemed safe enough to the xenotransplant community.

But that didn't sit right to one Brit by the name of Robin Weiss. Weiss was a world-famous virologist, focusing primarily on retroviruses—a type of virus that carries RNA rather than DNA as its genetic material and often leads to cancers. It also carries with it an enzyme, reverse transcriptase, that converts its RNA into DNA, allowing the virus to then replicate in the infected host. The most famous retrovirus is HIV, although others have been identified that lead to cancer in human cells. One of Weiss's earliest discoveries, while still a graduate student in the 1970s, was identifying a retrovirus that had inserted its DNA into the genome of chickens, including the germ line cells, that could be passed down from generation to generation, sometimes termed an "endogenous virus."[9] What was novel about Weiss's findings was the idea that viral DNA that was passed through generations could cause cancer in progeny, potentially generations after the DNA was inserted. He was fascinated by this concept, and also by the mechanisms of retroviral infections and their potential role in cancer. He decided to devote his entire career to their study.

Weiss's biggest discovery, however, was the identification of the receptor on T cells that the HIV virus uses to enter the cells and cause infection (the CD4 receptor), which he published in *Nature* in 1984.[10] A major portion of his career was devoted to the study of HIV (a zoonotic virus, not an endogenous virus).

He never lost his interest, however, in these endogenous viruses that could embed themselves in the DNA of the host and be passed down between generations.[11] They can also be considered evolutionarily advantageous as over time viruses have embedded into the human genome and supplied genes that have benefitted our species, including by giving us the ability to make placentas.[12] Weiss elaborated on the topic of the endogenous viruses in a speech he gave to the American Philosophical Society.[13] "When the germ line—the cells destined to become eggs or sperm—integrate viral DNA, the latent virus gains a free ride to the next generation, and to countless further generations through being inherited by the host as a Mendelian trait. We call these viral genomes endogenous retroviruses.[14] This phenomenon has occurred in all vertebrate species studied; for example, thanks to the complete sequencing of the human genome we now realize that approximately 8% of our DNA represents the paleontological record of germ line infection."

This represents a novel way to understand evolution and the role that viruses have played in helping humans evolve, while also keeping the viral DNA "alive" as free riders in the human genome. But why would a researcher focusing on human disease and particularly cancer be so intrigued by endogenous (or fossil) DNA? Weiss gave the following explanation in this same speech: "Such a collection of fossils would be of no medical concern if they were truly dead relics, as almost all of the human endogenous retroviral genomes appear to be. But some of the endogenous retroviruses have maintained the capacity to awake, Rip van Winkle-like, and to emerge again as infectious agents." In other words, portions of DNA inserted from a viral genome can lay dormant for generations, and then suddenly become relevant when transmitted to a new species or inserted into a novel genome.

In 1995, a couple of prominent virus researchers wrote a letter to *Nature Medicine* titled "The Dangers of Xenotransplantation."[15] In the article, the authors lamented the lack of concern that had been exhibited in relation to the potential risk of activation of endogenous viruses in xenotransplantation. Unlike other infections (bacteria and viruses) that could be screened for and potentially eliminated in clean herds, the endogenous viruses were embedded in the DNA of all pigs and could not be eliminated. Pigs, like all mammals, were known to harbor such viruses, termed PERVs. "Even the slightest trace of such a virus renders vector preparations absolutely unsafe for gene therapy trials; to casually ignore its virtual certain presence in transplant trials makes little sense."

This article resounded with Weiss. He and his team conducted a number of simple studies to assess the potential of cells of porcine origin to transmit the endogenous PERV virus to human cells. Their experiments were conducted with cell lines derived from pigs and humans, and they also analyzed cells harvested directly from various pig organs. They found that PERV was indeed produced and viral products, including active reverse transcriptase, could be demonstrated in the serum surrounding the pig-derived cells. They also identified that in certain conditions, cells from a human kidney cell line could become infected when exposed to the serum with virus that had been produced by the pig cell lines. It was previously known that human serum had the ability to lyse the viral vectors with the help of complement, possibly because the PERV virus picks up Alpha Gal when it is transcribed and liberated from pig cells. Weiss showed that once the virus was made in the human cell line, human serum and complement no longer had efficacy on the now human-generated virus. He further theorized that if the pig donor was ultimately an Alpha Gal knockout pig, this could remove a target that the human immune system would normally utilize to fight off this virus. Weiss further proposed that it is possible the reason humans and old-world monkeys have evolved to have natural antibody like Alpha Gal against other animals is to protect against pandemics caused by such endogenous bacteria and retroviruses as PERV. Genetic knockouts of this sugar molecule, along with disruption of the complement pathway, may be the perfect storm to allow these viruses to run rampant in human hosts.

Weiss published this work in the premier journal *Nature Medicine* in March of 1997, under the title "Infection of human cells by an endogenous retrovirus of pigs."[16] The paper was accompanied by commentary from a famous virologist cautioning regulatory bodies worldwide, including the FDA, to tread cautiously in considering human trials in xenotransplantation. "These issues are of global concern and it would be prudent for all countries to responsibly act together to prevent the introduction of infectious diseases, because a new emerging pathogen has no regard for national borders."[17]

This short article, conducted entirely in cell culture, confirmed the potential that these deeply embedded and hidden endogenous viral DNA segments could replicate and infect human cells. Whether it would happen in a living animal or person was entirely unknown, and even if it did happen, whether it would lead to any disease state was unknowable. But the article dropped like a bomb on the xenotransplantation community. A majority of transplant researchers waved their hands, saying PERV was unlikely to cause a problem, this was all theoretical, these endogenous viruses were not significant. But the timing couldn't have been worse. With so much fear worldwide from the AIDS epidemic, the public health community urged a halt on any consideration of human trials. Virologists agreed, stating that while the risks might be low, they were more than theoretical, especially with an organ sitting in an immunosuppressed patient potentially for years. The FDA rapidly convened a workshop on the topic, and in October of 1997, placed all ongoing clinical trials on hold.

Multiple groups (including Novartis and scientists at Imutran and Immerge) began rapidly screening the blood of more than two hundred patients who had received live pig tissues around the world in various trials of cell therapy. A majority of these patients had either received an infusion of islet cells to treat diabetes or short term perfusion of their blood through a pig kidney or liver, but none of them had an actual pig organ sewn into their bodies. With very sensitive PCR testing, none of those patients were found to have any evidence of PERV in their blood.[18] But the numbers were small, they didn't have vascularized organs that had human blood coursing through them with every heartbeat, and a majority of patients weren't on immunosuppression. This was some consolation, but as Weiss himself explained when describing the infection of human xenografts in a mouse model by endogenous virus, the rate was only 1 percent. "Thus, there is no room for complacency over the possibility of human infection, because if a host endogenous virus can infect human xenografts transplanted into animals, surely animal xenografts could be a source of infection to the human host." He further cautioned that "HIV-1 took decades to get going as an epidemic infection, and there is evidence that zoonotic transfer of a coronavirus related to SARS has occurred frequently among civet cat handlers, but has spread alarmingly from person to person on only one occasion thus far. Accordingly we must remain vigilant . . ."[19]

Members of the xenotransplant community tried to press on with their research. Industrial leaders were more shaken—what could be worse for a company making a major investment, in the hundreds of millions of dollars, than the prospect of unleashing a viral pandemic? Even a hint of such a thing, the smallest signal on a PCR assay of a single recipient, would send stock prices to the floor and lawyers into a frenzy. Whispers of contingency plans and cutting of losses were audible in boardrooms across the world.

* * * * *

The nail in the coffin came from one of the premier transplant researchers in the world, Fritz Bach. He was a giant in transplant immunology, who was one of the first people to understand the cellular basis of incompatibility and organ rejection. Bach remains one of the most colorful, controversial, and polarizing figures in transplantation. Early in his research career, he developed an assay using cells from a potential recipient and donor that might predict if a transplant could be conducted without rejection, an assay some have referred to as a transplant in a dish.[20] It is still used in immunology laboratories to this day. He was one of the first two people to successfully conduct a bone marrow transplant in a human in 1968, using his assay to predict the transplant would be accepted.[21] Bach extended this assay to use in organ transplantation, and it served as a foundation for clinical transplantation. He was on the short list for a Nobel Prize for this work, and many feel he deserved it. His career took him from Wisconsin to Minnesota to New York and finally back to Harvard, where he went to college and medical school. At every stop, Bach built large and productive labs and clinical programs, where he would directly translate his science into his medical practice. He was also an extraordinarily dynamic speaker and inspired many young researchers to devote themselves to the field of transplantation. He mentored many current leaders in immunology, who speak about him with the utmost respect.

At the same time, Bach was extremely competitive and egotistical, characteristics that ultimately left him isolated with a long list of enemies. To this day, when you ask anyone to describe their feelings regarding Bach the person, they will either say he was the most brilliant and inspirational person they have ever met, or that he was a narcissist who took the air out of the room whenever he entered.

The second half of Bach's career was focused entirely on xenotransplantation. He knew the barriers to immunologic success were massive, but he also thought they were surmountable. He and David Sachs shared this optimism and self-assuredness, and although their personalities were quite different, they became close friends. Bach's work, in cellular assays and animal models, was central to understanding the mechanisms of xenotransplant rejection, from hyperacute rejection with antibody, to the role of complement, to the powerful T cell responses that occurred if hyperacute rejection was avoided. David White's own work was based significantly on Bach's findings. But as White was regaling the press and the transplant community with his successes and predictions that trials were right around the corner, Bach was becoming more negative about the potential for White's transgenic pigs to succeed.

After Weiss's bombshell article on PERV was published in *Nature*, the majority of the transplant community was trying to craft a response that included caution and concern, but at the same time optimism that a path forward could be navigated. Xeno leaders like Sachs, Ayares, and White all agreed that the PERV data was concerning, but were relieved to discover that no humans exposed to pig cells had generated the virus, and were finding the same results in all the primates that received pig organs. Caution would be the word of the day, but if graft survival reached the milestones of six-month survival in primates, trials could proceed as long as recipients received appropriate informed consent and were monitored closely for any signs of the virus. The community was speaking with one voice on this topic, in discussions at transplant meetings, in scientific journals, and in the press.

Out of nowhere, in February of 1998, Bach dropped his own bomb. He published a commentary in *Nature Medicine* titled "Uncertainty in xenotransplantation: Individual benefit versus collective risk."[22] The article had a banner at the top with the following declaration, highlighted in pink: "Xenotransplantation continues to present daunting scientific hurdles but there is now a genuine prospect for clinical application. There are also significant and unknown risks. We call for a moratorium on all human xenotransplantation and offer a strategy for balancing the ethical, medical, scientific and societal demands of xenotransplantation prior to human clinical trials."

The article highlighted that genetically modified pig organs might serve as a threat to both humans and pigs for generations to come. Bach noted that the FDA had established an advisory committee including experts and lay representatives, but he did not believe this had gone far enough. He proposed a national committee with members from all walks of life to develop a consensus about whether it is worth proceeding with xenotransplantation, or "whether these efforts should be abandoned." He described xenotransplantation as the inverse of immunization. "Immunization is intended to protect the population at the risk of having occasional individuals experience adverse reactions to the immunization. Xenotransplantation, on the other hand, offers potential benefit to the individual while putting the population at risk." He wrote eloquently about the risk to pigs, related to animal rights, genetic manipulation, and the risk of causing an infection that could wipe out large pig populations. He explained that in assessing what the risk of a massive xenozoonosis (or infection caused by xenotransplantation) might be, "there are essentially no data which could be used accurately to assess the level of such risk. The range of uncertainty is large, with the possibility of devastating cross-species infection looming in the background."

Bach followed the publication of the article with a media blitz, including an appearance on *Fresh Air with Terry Gross* on February 17, 1998. He highlighted the potential that xenotransplantation would be putting the worldwide population at infectious risk. He explained that any fears that individuals in the population may have would be rational. When Terry asked him how great the risk was of a new epidemic, he responded "nobody can give you an answer to that, and I'm not going to even try. I can tell you the risk is greater than zero. There is a risk. . . . If it occurs, it is an awful event to happen." Towards the end of the interview, Terry mentioned that she found it interesting that he was so committed to xenotransplantation as a researcher and yet was leading the charge in calling for a moratorium. She asked him if he felt personally responsible for the potential risk xenotransplantation may cause to the general population. Bach agreed with that sentiment. "It is very important for those of us that have the privilege of doing biomedical research, and we really do lead a privileged life, to balance our concern for the patients, with being very responsible with what we do." Terry then asked him what the turning point was that led him to call for the moratorium. He answered that the turning point was that "a man in England, David White from a biotech company known as Imutran, said he was ready to do pig heart transplants to humans, and I thought that was so premature and to some extent irresponsible, and I came back and said, my heavens we have to really consider what we are doing here . . ." At the end of the interview, Bach highlighted that he was driven by the concept of Primum Non Nocere—Do No Harm.

The reaction in the xenotransplant community was one of horror. Everyone agreed that the risks needed to be taken seriously, and that patients needed to be closely monitored. But placing a moratorium on trials, creating committees, involving the public—this would extinguish all the momentum that was building in the transplant world. David Sachs responded with his own letter to *Nature Medicine*.[23] In the letter, Sachs highlighted that the FDA already had convened a committee that included national leaders and members of the lay public to discuss these issues related to xenotransplantation. He stressed that "the halting of a medical practice for which risk has not yet been assessed would create a dangerous precedent. In fact, there is no way to assess that risk adequately without such clinical trials." He discussed that many other trials had the potential to affect public health, including the use of novel antibiotics that ran the risk of selecting bacteria that were more and more resistant to available therapies, and it was the FDA that regulated those trials. He ended the letter with the statement that "we therefore think it important to clarify that not all members of the transplantation community back the call for a moratorium on well-controlled, clinical research on xenotransplantation."

The FDA made a decision to put all clinical trials in humans on hold, declaring that in the future they would need to approve any future trials, rather than leave it up to local IRBs and hospital ethics committees. This applied to any living pig trials in humans, from cell therapy to *ex-vivo* organ perfusions to organ transplants. In the Unitd Kingdom, a strong moratorium was placed on all proposed xenotransplantation trials. Industry leaders attacked the call for a moratorium. The head of research and development for Novartis, Paul Herrling, was quoted as saying "Animals have transmitted viruses to humans throughout history. The added risk of xenotransplantation might be minimal."[24]

Between the numerous protests of animal rights activists in the United Kingdom, now energized by reports of the risks of a massive pandemic that xeno could cause and the strong reaction of the UK Xenotransplantation Interim Regulatory Authority, the writing was on the wall regarding the future of xeno in the United Kingdom. The fear that mad cow disease had caused was still fresh in the mind of every Brit, and the UK government was not going to take any chances regarding another animal-derived illness. Within two years, Imutran would cease to exist. Xenotransplantation would be all but dead in the UK, never to recover to this day. Even as Novartis announced its shift of investment to the United States, the leadership of Novartis began discussions on an exit plan from the discipline entirely. By the time the first pigs were cloned Virginia, and the Alpha Gal knockout was nearing reality, the ultimatum had already been given to the Davids by both Novartis and PPL: unless you solve the barriers to clinical xenotransplantation in the next year, there will be no more industrial support.

Why didn't Bach think it was enough to simply call for caution, to research the risk of PERV and other sources of infection without calling for an immediate and absolute moratorium? If you ask xeno-researchers from that era who are still around today, they call Bach an attention-seeker. They say he was jealous that White was receiving so much press and always delivered the keynote talk at every transplant conference. Bach couldn't stand to see people grandstanding about their incredible results and being described in the press as the pioneers when so much of their work was based on his own discoveries.

But perhaps it was something else. Bach was born in Vienna, Austria in 1934, and after Kristallnacht, he and his brother were sent to England through the Kinder Transport program that saved ten thousand Jewish children in Europe. Maybe Bach's experience as a child, watching a totalitarian government indiscriminately kill half its own population, forcing him to be shipped out of the country in the dead of night without most of his family weighed on him. Much of his own family was killed, although his brother and parents survived by fleeing to the United States. Perhaps this gave Bach a sense of responsibility to protect the public from a horrible pandemic that could indiscriminately kill them. Maybe the idea that a few prominent researchers and government officials could make a decision that would affect millions of helpless men, women, and children was too much for Bach to bear. He may have had a natural and inbred distrust that authority would protect the masses.

Bach remained a pariah in the transplant community for the rest of his career. He continued to conduct research, present at meetings, and teach students. But he will be most remembered in the xenotransplant community as the man who almost destroyed the field forever. Bach died on August 14, 2011, at his home, virtually alone. At the time of his death, xenotransplantation remained what it was in 1998—a purely scientific endeavor. The moratorium was still in place.

Robin Weiss, the person who opened Pandora's box and warned the world of the potential risk of PERV, himself a great admirer of Bach's courageous call for a moratorium, deserves one last word on the topic.

"Thus there is much to ponder on the ethics and safety of xenotransplantation. Will society regard xenotransplant recipients as dangerous lepers and demand that they live in quarantine? For how long after xenotransplantation will they need to be monitored for infection? Can one require that their intimate partners also be tested for porcine infection? To what extent should the precautionary principle override the opportunity to make progress in medicine through advancing technologies? While surgeons tend to weigh concern about the infection hazard in xenotransplantation as a risk-benefit equation calculated for the individual patient, it behooves us to take the broader view and attempt to balance risk-benefit to the community at large. Although the likelihood of epidemic spread of a porcine virus appears even more remote than an individual patient's acquiring infection, the consequences would be more drastic. Surely we need a Hippocratic oath for public health that would minimize harm to the community resulting from the treatment of individuals? Overall, one can sum up xenotransplantation with the same aphorism that Joshua Lederberg applied to the debate on recombinant DNA technology at Asilomar nearly thirty years ago: it holds certain promise and uncertain peril."[25]

* * * * *

When PPL leadership looked at the landscape for xenotransplantation, it was hard to be optimistic. They recognized that Ayares and his team were rapidly making progress. But being based in the United Kingdom, what they really saw were massive protests, some violent, against the proposals to breed animals for human organs. Novartis was in the process of pulling the plug on Imutran, and although it still had a three-year commitment to a US company, it was clear that the company's interest in xeno was waning. If that wasn't enough, the idea of unleashing a global pandemic into the world squashed any remaining interest in the field. The horrendous experience with mad cow disease, highlighted daily by stories on the evening news and across the front page of every newspaper showing young people losing the ability to walk, feed themselves, talk, and suffering painful deaths left British society terrified by idea of a xenovirus. The UK Xenotransplantation Interim Regulatory Authority had removed any possibility of a xenotransplant clinical trial in the future, so the only hope for a trial was across the pond.

As early as 2000, Ayares got word that he was going to have to raise money to sustain his xeno efforts, as PPL had serious interest in divesting from the Virginia subsidiary. Ayares used those two years as a crash course in fundraising and leadership. He knew he was competing head-to-head with David Sachs and his collaborators at BioTransplant, soon to become Immerge with the backing of Novartis. He also knew that Sachs, an academic through and through, would be publishing his results in the best scientific journals after lengthy peer review, shunning flashy announcements in the press, at least until after the articles were published. Ayares was aware that once a peer-reviewed paper was accepted into a major journal, the investigators had to agree to an embargo on releasing any information about the findings until after the paper was posted online. Given how closely the two teams were progressing, Ayares decided to delay publication until after his press releases, and with each announcement, he would highlight how PPL was at the forefront in generating transgenic pigs. He was sure to reiterate that there were no more barriers to clinical xenotransplantation, and always to make a reference to PPL's role in the cloning of Dolly the sheep. Ayares was aware that many members of the scientific community would look down on him for this strategy, but he didn't care. He needed the money to keep his company alive.

By early 2002, shortly after the announcement that the single knockout pigs existed and the team was working feverishly at cloning or breeding double knockouts, Ayares got word that PPL was in the process of downsizing and would be facing bankruptcy in the near future. Ayares had six months to spin off his Virginia division as a new company, or the doors would be shuttered. He spent the next six months giving presentations to venture capital funds, pharmaceutical companies, banks, and anyone who had any money and a little time. Ayares gave more than seventy presentations to venture capital funds alone, to no avail. The number one concern voiced to Ayares during these presentations was PERV and the risk of causing a pandemic. The science was great, but who wanted to take that kind of risk? It didn't help that his presentations coincided with the bursting of the dot-com bubble, and a concurrent stock market crash. Ayares traveled all over the United States, Canada, and then the world, going as far as China, and came up with nothing. The pharmaceutical market was an absolute nonstarter. Novartis was in the process of pulling out of xeno, and Baxter was already out.

Ayares turned to the one person he thought might be able to help him—Starzl. Ayares told Starzl they had recently birthed the Alpha Gal double knockouts, but he was out of money. PPL was going under, and Ayares with it. Starzl was not going to let that happen. He first reached out to a group in Saudi Arabia where he had close connections. In 1983, Starzl performed a kidney transplant on Princess Sultana, a member of the house of Saud and one of the King's many children. In late 2002, after Starzl's phone call, a group from the country was considering an investment to buy the Virginia PPL subsidiary. At the last minute, the Grand Mufti weighed in and forbade it, proclaiming it would go against Muslim law to support a company seeking to use pigs as organ donors for humans.

Starzl next reached out to Fujisawa (now named Astellas Pharma), the large Japanese pharmaceutical company that had developed tacrolimus with Starzl, the blockbuster drug that ultimately would replace cyclosporine. Starzl had single-handedly rescued this drug from oblivion and made the company billions of dollars with no personal gain. But Fujisawa had no interest in being a lead investor in a xenotransplantation company in 2002, knockout pig or not. They would consider a smaller investment if someone else took the lead.

At the beginning of 2003, Ayares met with Starzl in his office in Pittsburgh and told him he had struck out everywhere. PPL had given Ayares the notification that it was finally cutting ties. Ayares wondered if Starzl knew of any jobs for an experienced, soon-to-be-unemployed gene editor. Starzl wouldn't hear it. He had one more card to play. The University of Pittsburgh had a sizable venture fund, with much of its endowment coming from the profits of the very transplant center he had started and run for a decade, the Thomas E. Starzl Transplantation Institute. He did not think Pittsburgh would buy the company outright, but figured he may be able to talk them into being the lead investor if Fujisawa would join the group. Starzl accompanied Ayares to the pitch meetings, no doubt influencing the outcome with his larger-than-life presence in the boardroom. After multiple presentations, the University of Pittsburgh venture fund agreed to be the lead investor, along with Fujisawa and Highmark Health Ventures Investment Fund of Pittsburgh. PPL, which was desperate to part with the Blacksburg subsidiary, agreed to sell it off for the low price of $3.5 million. In April of 2003, the Blacksburg subsidiary became Revivicor, and David Ayares was the CEO. Money was still tight, but they were alive, and so was the Alpha Gal knockout.

* * * * *

Back in the Charlestown Navy Yard, experiments using Goldie's organs began in February of 2003. The surgical teams that performed the transplants were led by Yamada (renal transplants) and Cooper (heart transplants). Goldie's donation took place on Wednesday, February 19. Sachs tried to go about his day like any other, but his mind was racing and he couldn't stay focused. All he wanted to do was sit in the operating room and watch his teams work.

After Goldie's chest and abdomen were opened, Yamada removed the thymus and both kidneys. He would perform a vascularized thymus transplant and kidney transplant into one baboon recipient. Yamada would first remove that baboon's own thymus, sewing the pig thymus into that same space. Once this was complete, he would open the baboon's belly, remove its spleen and both its kidneys, and then perform a kidney transplant using one of Goldie's kidneys. He would then close this baboon, and while he was doing this, his team of technicians would be prepping another baboon in the room next door. Yamada would then transplant Goldie's other kidney into that baboon without the thymus, as a control for the importance of the thymus transplant.

Once Yamada had his organs out, Cooper's team would move in. He removed Goldie's heart, ending her short life, while his team was prepping a baboon recipient. Once he had Goldie's heart in bowl, flushed of all its blood and sitting lifeless on ice, he would open the baboon's belly and sew the heart onto the aorta and cava; after releasing the clamps, the heart would start beating. This was a heterotopic heart, which would beat but not be life sustaining—the baboon would keep its own heart for that.

February 19 went perfectly, and there were many more days like it. Yamada, Cooper, and everyone in the lab worked like they were possessed over the next eighteen months. As soon as more knockout pigs were available, transplants were performed. Everything had to be coordinated so no precious organs were wasted. Team members were at the lab day and night, either preparing for new transplants or sitting in the baboon room taking care of the recipients. After the transplants, blood collected from the recipients would be used in assays, mixed with blood that had been collected and frozen from the donors. The presence of any antibody in the baboon blood was analyzed, and the activity of baboon immune cells was tested, using versions of the "transplant in a test tube" assay that Fritz Bach had devised three decades before. Baboons were surviving longer than ever before, and the assays were confirming that their cells were less responsive, less angry at the pig donors. But every time a baboon recipient died, or a graft petered out, it was like they lost one of their best friends. A pall of darkness would settle over the lab as the dying baboons were brought to the operating room to remove their transplants and other tissues for analysis.

By mid-2004, the teams were writing up their results, which were published in two separate *Nature Medicine* papers posted online December 26. In the report on kidney transplants, Yamada and his team described eleven transplants of kidney and thymus, five of which were thymokidneys and six as vascularized thymic lobes.[26] Three kidneys were transplanted without any thymus. The recipients received a variety of immunosuppression protocols that included removing their spleens, giving them antibodies to deplete their T cells, steroids, strong maintenance immunosuppression, and some pre-treated with radiation. Three of the vascularized thymic lobe recipients died early from technical causes, but the three that made it through the protocol kept their grafts for 31, 56, and 68 days. The two thymokidney recipients that made it through the protocol lasted 81 and 83 days. The three kidneys from the Alpha Gal knockouts transplanted without thymus lasted 20, 33, and 34 days before they were rejected.

In Cooper's report, eight Alpha Gal knockout hearts were transplanted, and two control hearts with Gal served as controls.[27] Five of the eight knockouts made it through the protocol. The knockout heart graft survival ranged from 59 to 179 days, with a mean of 99 days. The two controls were rejected within twenty minutes of implant.

At the end of Yamada's paper, the authors summarized their findings. They considered the results encouraging and highlighted that no previous pig-to-primate kidney transplant had survived so long.

Still, the grafts failed. None of them achieved a survival of six months, the minimum that would be required to justify moving into human trials. There was more work to be done. That's how science always works.

But more work would mean more money, and that was in short supply. Novartis reached the end of its three-year commitment in early 2003, just as the knockout experiments were starting. Paul Herrling, the head of research, was incredulous that after the $100 million investment in xeno, returns could be expected anytime soon. "The results, while extremely interesting from a scientific point of view, were still not close enough to a practical application.

We are not a university who is doing science for science's sake—we need at the end of the day when we invest to have a product coming out of it."[28]

In the fall of 2003, Herrling let Sachs and the leadership of Immerge know Novartis was officially pulling the plug on its investment. As for the early results Immerge was reporting from the knockouts, Herrling said the following. "It was a step in the right direction, but in practical terms, it did not significantly change the equation." Novartis was out.

The leadership at Immerge engaged in the same process that Ayares had just a year earlier, presenting results and business plans to venture capital firms, banks, medical/pharma companies, anyone who would listen. But no one would bite. Sachs was writing grants to every agency he could think of, but running the xeno experiments was just too expensive to sustain solely on government grants. Although he could conceivably get funding to analyze mechanisms of rejection, it was unlikely the government would fund the generation of new transgenic pigs. That was the kind of thing industry had to pay for.

Sachs found himself deeply frustrated, at a time when the science was more exciting than ever. "My major concern right now is not whether the biology and the immunology are capable of overcoming the rest of the problems. It's whether or not we're going to be able to continue to get sufficient funding for these studies. It's more of a worry to me now than the biology, which is a very unusual place for me because it's the first time the actual results are anywhere near this encouraging—and yet it's also the first time when the funding situation has looked so critical."[29]

By spring of 2004, as Yamada and Cooper were writing up their results furiously, and Sachs was doing the same with grant applications, Immerge Biotherapeutics was running on fumes. They essentially had no full-time employees or even an office. Immerge was a website with some IP that no one wanted. Experiments on the knockouts had dwindled down to a trickle, as they just didn't have enough pigs. Sachs focused on breeding the ones he had rather than using them for experiments, and risk losing the entire line of double knockouts.

In early 2004, Cooper met with Sachs and let him know that he had gotten a call from Starzl informing him that Starzl and Ayares were looking for someone to run their efforts with xenotransplantation at Pittsburgh, utilizing the pigs from the now fully funded Revivicor. Cooper didn't want to leave Sachs, but his obsession remained making xenotransplantation a reality. The writing was on the wall in the Sachs lab. No more transgenic pigs were going to be cloned, and it was just a matter of time before they would run out of the knockouts entirely.

By mid-year, Cooper would leave Boston, and by the time their Alpha Gal knockout paper was published, Cooper was already listed at the Starzl Transplantation Institute. Sachs understood Cooper's move, and although he was sad to see him go, he supported his longtime friend. More than anything Sachs wanted to see xenotransplantation succeed, and in his lifetime. The thing that kept him up at night, that bothered him when he would allow the thoughts to enter his head, is that he might die and not get to see how this would all play out. "I don't resent the fact that there's so much we don't know," he said. "In fact, I'm awed by it. What I resent is the fact that I won't be around to see the things understood that I want to understand and to see the answers. It makes me sad. And the older I get, the sadder it makes me."[30]

Sachs was not going to sit back and throw in the towel. He would keep his work going. If industry wouldn't fund it, he would write even more grants. He would keep working on his two major strategies in the xeno model—bone marrow transplants to establish mixed chimerism, and thymus transplant. He had some other ideas about new gene edits in pigs, maybe adding a gene or two to reduce the immune response to allow engraftment of cells or organs. But these new edits would need to wait. For now, Sachs would focus on breeding up the pigs he already had. There was plenty to do with them.

* * * * *

While Sachs and his team were proceeding with the double-knockout transplants, Ayares was already thinking about what other genes he should manipulate to make the pig a better organ donor for humans. Starzl had predicted that the Alpha Gal knockout would be enough, that they would be able to move rapidly through primate experiments into human trials. He had wanted to get xeno back into humans ever since he had performed the two baboon liver transplants in humans ten years earlier. At that time, he had approval from Pittsburgh to perform more of them, but had decided there was no point. "Our whole investigative team is working on almost nothing except xenotransplantation," Starzl told *The Scientist* in August 1995.[31] "So, perhaps we have a strong insight about how tough this really is. We're not going to open up again until we have something that we think is a very fundamental improvement. Even though we've had permission to go forward, we're not nuts."

Starzl was convinced the Alpha Gal knockout was a very fundamental improvement. Sachs and his team wondered if Starzl would go right into humans. But Starzl initially had another plan, something in between a monkey and a living human. The University of Pittsburgh had formed a committee, termed "The Committee for Oversight of Research Involving the Dead," that would evaluate research projects aimed at trialing medications and devices in patients declared brain dead.[32] This wasn't a new concept, as a number of researchers had previously tried drugs, devices, and even an artificial heart in brain dead patients. As one member of the ethics committee at Pittsburgh said, "From a pure science point of view, this is just too good a research population to ignore."[33]

Despite the approval, Starzl ultimately decided not to do this. The results their group obtained using Revivicor's Alpha Gal knockout pigs in primates were much worse than he expected, even worse than the outcomes obtained in the Sachs lab. Their recipients only survived a few weeks. Starzl was disappointed and surprised. Ayares was not. Approaching the xeno challenge as a geneticist rather than a transplant surgeon, he always assumed that once Gal was taken care of, there would be more genes he would need to deal with. Whereas Starzl and others in the transplant world would focus on immunosuppression they might have to add, it was natural for Ayares to think of what other genes they would need to target.

So right after Revivicor was established, Ayares began searching for his next genetic target. He settled on one of the complement regulatory genes similar to those White had focused on. He reached out to an Australian company that had already made a pig with this gene inserted, and he bought the pigs and the rights to the IP. Once they arrived, he would start breeding them to his Alpha Gal knockout. He figured each new gene he added or subtracted might chip away at the pig-to-primate barrier, adding weeks or months of survival. Like Sachs, Ayares would never consider giving up on xeno. He knew they would get there eventually. Unlike Sachs, Ayares was in a vaguely more favorable situation financially, at least for the moment. He knew that wouldn't last forever.

With Starzl approaching eighty years old, both he and Ayares agreed they needed someone else to run their efforts in the lab, someone who had experience transplanting pig organs into primates. What better place to look than in Sachs's lab, their main competitor. They reached out to David Cooper shortly after Novartis had pulled the plug on Immerge. They told Cooper they had a commitment from the University of Pittsburgh to fund Revivicor for a while—not for the long term, but at least the "medium term." That was enough for Cooper. He knew he couldn't do better than that.

6 THE XENO-VISIONARIES OF THE TWENTY-FIRST CENTURY

With the loss of industry funding, concerns over PERV, and protests from animal rights activists, xenotransplantation retreated back into the woodwork. The research in pre-clinical models continued, funded almost entirely by government grants. Presentations on xeno were relegated to breakout sessions and early morning symposiums at national transplant meetings. But the spark of promise that xeno would one day become a reality was not entirely extinguished. What the field needed was a new, modern set of visionaries who were willing to devote their reputations, their lives, to the field. They each needed to be driven by something personal that would never let them accept failure or fear success. These innovators, we'll call them "xeno-visionaries," needed to believe, to just know, that xeno would become a reality in their lifetime. And they needed to be in a position to harness the novel, earth-shattering advances in gene editing that were rapidly gripping the imagination of every scientist, venture capitalist, and journalist coming of age in the early part of the twenty-first century. These scientific innovations would serve as the kindling for the revolution that would be xeno. These visionaries will be the ones to ignite the flames.

————

"This is an extremely rare disease. No one knows why it arises."

She listened.

"There are no medicines approved for it. . . . All the patients die within two to three years.

What can you do?

"All you can do is hope for a lung transplant."

That seemed like terrible news. But the next piece of information was even worse. The head of pediatric cardiology at Children's National Hospital in Washington, DC, one of the most famous and experienced pediatric specialists in the world, had only taken care of three children with this diagnosis. All three had died.

"I was crushed. I just saw black."[1]

This could not be happening, Martine thought. Just a few years ago, Jenesis had been a normal, healthy little girl, the youngest of four that Martine and her wife Bina shared. But on a recent trip to Telluride, they had noticed that Jenesis couldn't keep up with her siblings. She took on an almost blue tint in the high altitude of Colorado and struggled to breathe. When they returned home to Maryland, she appeared better but continued to complain that she was always tired. They brought her to countless doctors, who prescribed inhalers and said Jenesis had asthma or was just out of shape. Then came the random fainting. "I'd start to hear something like the tinkling of fairy dust, if that makes any sense. Then I'd see little dark spots, going from the outside in, until it was one big black spot."[2]

Then she would faint, dropping as if shot.

By 1994, Jenesis would struggle walking up the few steps to her bedroom at the end of the day. It was then, at Children's National Hospital in Washington, DC, that Jenesis was finally given a diagnosis. She had primary pulmonary hypertension (PPH), a disease that was untreatable and usually fatal.

Martine had recently turned forty years old, but in many ways, her life had just begun. She had spent the last two decades chasing a vision that had come to her while penniless on a beach in Seychelles, a dream that any normal person would have thought was impossible. Yet she had done it, she had navigated the far reaches of space itself. As if that wasn't enough, she was in the midst of her own rebirth, the new beginning of the rest of her life. Although she was assigned male at birth, she had known that she was female since her early teens, if not earlier. She was well on her way to becoming the person she had always known she was. Yet now, her youngest child, her Jenesis, was given a death sentence. There was nothing she could do. But that was not how Martine approached the world. She wasn't like other people.

There was always something she could do. "I felt like my only purpose in life now was not to help move to the stars with satellites and stuff like that. It was to save Jenesis. So I just stopped everything I was doing."[3] So what was it she was doing anyways?

* * * * *

Martine Rothblatt was born in 1954 in Chicago, Illinois, and soon after the family relocated to San Diego, California where her father Harold would run a dental practice. Martine's childhood was what you might describe as "normal" and "safe," although hers was the only Jewish family in a Hispanic neighborhood. She embraced this idea of being different, and from an early age was always trying to learn about different cultures and ways of life, both in social interactions and in the books she would read. Astronomy and space captivated her from an early age, and the idea of living amongst the celestial stars became a recurring dream for Martine.

Martine enrolled in UCLA in the early 1970s with a love of the stars in the sky above her, but no real idea about what that might mean for her life. She had hoped that when she entered college, she would quickly identify some greater meaning for her life, some academic path that would grasp her imagination and allow her to find purpose. Instead, she found herself listless and unmotivated. After sophomore year, Martine dropped out of college to see the world and to find her place in it.

Martine started in Europe, then went to the Middle East, and then to East Africa, and in the summer of 1974 found herself in the islands of Seychelles. Seychelles was inherently beautiful, but her accommodations were decidedly not, complete with cockroaches and locusts. By chance, Martine scored an invite to the Indian Ocean Station, a US Air Force Satellite Control Network tracking station based in Seychelles. As Martine travelled up La Misere Road, a gigantic, beautiful golf ball came into view. It wasn't a ball, of course, but a radome that housed the sixty-foot antenna used to contact and receive messages from the satellites coursing along their orbits over the Indian Ocean.

Martine gazed in awe at the big satellite dish. "It was like we stepped into the future. Everything was crisp and clean. It seemed to me the satellite engineer was making the whole world come together. Like that was the center of the world."[4] Martine began speaking excitedly to the engineer, wanting to understand everything this satellite was capable of. She couldn't believe it was possible to send a message into outer space that would arrive at a satellite spaceship in orbit, and she was even more stunned that this same satellite could accurately send signals back to the station where they were standing.

A vision started to form in her head. She peppered the engineer with questions, which he happily answered, excited to have a captive audience to break the monotony of his lonely existence. Eventually Martine asked him the question that had been marinating in her brain since she first saw the giant dish housed in the golf ball. Would it ever be possible to send signals from a satellite in orbit down to individual people, if they each had their own small dish? Perhaps, for instance, a dish mounted in their house, or maybe even on their car? The engineer thought about it for a moment. It could be possible, he said, if the satellite was big enough, powerful enough. Martine was flabbergasted. "I fell in love and was intoxicated by satellite communications. It seemed magical that we can put a machine way out in space and it can do amazing things across the planet."[5]

She experienced an epiphany that almost knocked her off her feet. "That's the purpose of my life." "You can get this kind of excitement at any point in life. I think the best way to describe it would be a lightning bolt to your soul."[6]

Martine rushed back to UCLA and re-enrolled. She majored in communications studies, learning the engineering behind satellite technology and rounding out her education with classes on astronomy. Her senior thesis was on international direct-broadcast satellites, and she graduated *summa cum laude* in 1977. By this point Martine was forming some specific ideas about her vision for the future, connecting satellites to everyday people around the world. She knew she needed a better understanding of the complexities of the satellite business and the regulations that were just being put in place in the industry. She enrolled in the four-year joint business and law degree program at UCLA.

* * * * *

It was during Martine's graduate studies, years before her transition, that she first laid eyes on Bina (full name Beverlee), at a networking event in Hollywood. "I saw Bina sitting over there, and I just felt an enormous attraction to her and just walked over and asked her to dance. And she agreed to dance. We danced, we sat down, talked, and we've been together ever since."[7] It was now the second time a lightning bolt struck Martine's soul. Martine describes that in the moment she saw an "aura of energy around" Bina. When Martine felt that lightning strike, identified an objective that she wanted to achieve, she would chase it with singular focus and unrelenting effort. "You've got to work on something that you have a passion for," Rothblatt said. "You've got to feel that the success of your project is even more important than your own life."[8] This applied to business pursuits and personal relationships. Thankfully, Bina saw the same aura of energy around Martine. They knew immediately that they would be together forever. Martine felt more complete than she ever had before.

Martine graduated with her JD and MBA in 1981, and joined a law firm in Washington, DC. Much of her time was spent representing television broadcasting companies in interactions with the Federal Communications Commission (FCC), the same regulatory body that has jurisdiction over satellite communications. She began developing connections in the regulatory industry that would become crucial for her future success. But Martine knew she wouldn't spend her life working for a big law firm representing the television industry; she wanted to launch satellites, big satellites that would reach everyone occupying Planet Earth. Then she wanted to go to space herself. "Satellites, to me, are like the canoes that our ancestors first pushed out into the water," which allow for "navigation of the oceans of the sky."[9] Most satellites were small at this point, primarily launched and managed by branches of the government and military. Martine wanted to launch bigger and more powerful satellites, allowing small receiving antennaes, so small that they could be placed on private offices, homes, and even cars. Most everyone in the industry thought this would be impossible. But not Martine. "You've got to be able to question authority and say, 'why can't this succeed? Why can't my product work? . . . You also have to be persistent, because there will be so many times that you just feel like giving up."[10]

The dream that Martine would never let go led her on a whirlwind tour of the burgeoning satellite industry, a tour that encompassed almost two decades of her life and took her from a naïve undergraduate with an idea to the founder and CEO of the most innovative and groundbreaking satellite company the world had ever seen.

In 1990, after serving as the CEO of a startup satellite company, Martine was finally ready to launch her own satellite company that could send strong signals from space to anyone who happened to have a receiver in their house or their car. When she first pitched her idea to anyone who would listen, she was greeted with raised eyebrows and doubters. But one thing Martine had learned in business school was how to pitch the value of her idea and show it would be worth so much more in the future. More than 90 percent of her potential investors said no. But that left the potential for 10 percent to say yes. "You will run into a believer if you don't give up. Never give up." Before long she had raised enough money to design and launch a few satellites. Martine convinced the FCC to license this new company as a subscription service rather than a typical radio service supported by advertisers. Subscribers would be able to listen to radio stations from anywhere in the United States at any time. She would approach every car dealership, company, rental agency in the country and convince them to subscribe. She further convinced the FCC to assign unused frequencies for satellite radio broadcast. Radio stations across the country were aghast. Sirius Satellite Radio was born, with Martine as CEO and Chairman of the Board. Subscriptions grew every year, and talent was soon knocking at the door to sign on. The company went public in 1994, and the company continued to see massive growth and lucrative earnings. Martine was rich.

* * * * *

In the early 1990s, Martine's business was thriving, and she was sought after for board positions, consulting contracts, and collaborations all across the satellite and communications industry. She was entirely comfortable pitching projects to CEOs and billionaires, convincing regulators why she should be allowed to transcend the terrestrial world of radio and get approval for broadcasting techniques they had never heard of, and ignoring the "naysayers and ankle biters" encountered at every turn. The doubters invigorated her. But she held one secret that left her more vulnerable, anxious, and insecure than anything she had ever encountered in a board room or at a podium. Martine knew, had known since the age of fifteen, that her soul was always female, even though her body was that of a man.

When she was young, Martine was afraid people would laugh at her, and she bottled those feelings up. Now in her late thirties, more than a decade after "finding herself" at an isolated satellite tracking station in the Seychelles, she was ready to finally be true to herself. But what would the one person she cared about more than anyone in the world think? Bina, her spice, the mother of her four children in their blended family—how would she react to the news? Her response was so simple, so obvious. "I love you for your soul, not your skin."

Martine then began the difficult task of telling her four children about her decision. She would become Martine, she would be identifying primarily as a woman, including in her dress, she would begin taking hormones, and eventually would undergo surgical reassignment. Each of the four children had a different reaction, but all were supportive. Their eldest son wondered what she was waiting for, "since we only live once and time keeps on ticking." Their seventeen-year-old daughter responded that "lots of people have two moms or two dads." Their eleven-year-old son asked: "Will you still be my dad?" "I'll still be your dad," Martine answered. "I'm not changing. I'm only changing physically. I'm going to be like a butterfly." Their youngest daughter Jenesis, then nine, considered being transgender "just another way people can be."

"And so began the years of transition. There were hormones, of course, and endless hours of psychotherapy aimed at establishing that Martine's urge was neither fleeting nor shallow. She began dressing as a woman in ever-widening circles—first out with Bina alone, then with friends, and finally on weekends with the kids and their friends. The children . . . agree it was an anguishing time. They were teased at school ("Who wears the pants in your family now?"); neighbors moved away."[11]

One arena where the transition didn't seem to jeopardize Martine was at work. Sirius was thriving. Regulators were approving Martine's well-honed proposals. Investors were lining up to be a part of this new technology. Collaborators were reaching out to Martine to see how she could help them with their own ventures. Martine reflected on this time years later: "Perhaps one investor summed up the hidden thoughts of many. He asked if it was true that I used to be a man. 'Yes,' I replied with a smile. 'Well,' he continued, 'I don't care if you walk around in a gorilla suit so long as you make as much money for me in the future as you did in the past.'"[12]

Martine saw her transition as another opportunity to push back on the arbitrary limits of society and challenge the ignorance that she encountered around her. She spent countless hours working on her "manifesto on the freedom of gender" titled *The Apartheid of Sex*, which would be published in 1995.[13] Martine wanted to be a role model—a supporter for the hundreds, thousands, maybe even millions of people that were struggling the way she once did. She was becoming an icon, a trailblazer in the world of business, space, and now gender. Even her name became iconic—Martine Rothblatt, like Madonna or Beyoncé, gradually became known by a single moniker: Martine. At this point, it's hard to imagine her being called anything else.

* * * * *

This was the position Martine found herself in when her beloved Jenesis received her terminal diagnosis in 1994. It was Jenesis who reminded Martine that she couldn't wait for someone else to take control of the situation. "'Martine was going through her transition and had been kind of considering retiring,' said Jenesis. 'I can remember crying myself to sleep many a night, thinking, *I don't want to die*. I remember thinking, *If you're going to be around the house all the time, then maybe you can do something to help me*.'"[14]

This hit Martine like another lightning bolt to her soul. But how could Martine save Jenesis? She had never heard of primary pulmonary hypertension (PPH). She hadn't taken a biology class since tenth grade! Most of the doctors whom Martine consulted themselves barely knew what this disease was. And the doctor had mentioned that Jenesis might need a lung transplant. Martine had no idea what that might entail. But she was going to find out.

The first thing Martine did was sell some shares of Sirius and use three million dollars to start the PPH Cure Foundation. She sponsored six-figure grants to researchers with proposals to treat the condition. She talked to doctors, researchers, and families that had been touched with the disease. Mostly, she read. Jenesis spent much of the early 1990s in hospitals, and Bina and Martine would take turns sleeping by her bedside. After Jenesis would fall asleep, Martine would head down to the stacks in the medical school library to conduct her research. If Jenesis was up to it, she would accompany Martine to the stacks. Martine describes the experience as "taking herself to school." She picked up where she had left off in the tenth grade, with high school biology and chemistry textbooks. Once she had a basic understanding of lung physiology, she acquired some college-level biology, anatomy, and chemistry textbooks. Then she started accessing scientific articles, anything that mentioned "primary pulmonary hypertension" or "pulmonary artery hypertension." As she read the articles, she constantly had to refer back to her textbooks to understand the text. She took notes, looked up words, read and re-read sections repeatedly. It slowly got easier. After a few months, she was reading articles straight through and understanding them fully. She studied the figures. At the end of each article, she would pull up the references and go back to the stacks and find them all. At first, the work seemed insurmountable, but eventually Martine noticed that in any given paper, she would already have read 90 percent of the references. She was becoming an expert.

Martine discovered much about the normal physiology of the lungs and circulatory system, but little about potential treatments for PPH. The only approved treatments for patients were the use of blood pressure medicines that dilated blood vessels—in particular calcium channel blockers. A small percentage of patients would respond to high-dose calcium channel blockers. But for those that didn't respond, there were no other approved treatments. The only drug under trial for advanced disease was called Flolan, made by the pharmaceutical company Glaxo. Flolan was a chemical substance found in the body that dilates blood vessels, and was shown in experimental protocols to have some efficacy in the treatment of PPH. It was only given to patients with severe heart failure accompanying the PPH, as it had to be administered intravenously, twenty-four hours per day, through a portable pump infused through a catheter permanently placed in the patient. That meant no showers, no swimming pools, no normal childhood. If Jenesis were to get sicker, that was what she had to look forward to. To Martine, the treatment seemed worse than the disease.

In early 1996, Martine reached out to James Crow, the pharmacologist who ran the research team that had developed Flolan while working at Burroughs Wellcome & Co. She had come across his name while reading an early paper on the development of the drug. She read everything Crow had ever published, including an obscure paper testing a molecule for the treatment of heart failure in a rat model of the disease. The molecule was unsuccessful, but she did notice one particular graph that showed a reduction in pulmonary pressure in the rats. Crow was retired by this point, living in North Carolina, and wasn't interested in rehashing his work with some aggressive business executive. Martine was relentless. She sent him email after email asking him about this molecule and whether it could be developed into a drug. His response was one word, capitalized: "NO." That wasn't a word Martine would accept. She began calling him every day. When she finally got a hold of him after Crow had dodged her calls for months, she demanded an in-person meeting. Crow told her he wasn't available. "'No,' she said. 'I've already got your ticket. I want to meet you in DC.'" Crow remembered her saying, "At the Four Seasons. On Thursday.'"[15]

When Crow did meet with Martine, he explained to her that Flolan was the only drug Glaxo would develop. He did remember the molecule in question and the work he did with it on rats. It had some unique properties, and Crow initially had great interest in this substance. While he was characterizing it, Burroughs Wellcome was bought by Glaxo and the two companies merged, becoming Glaxo Wellcome. Glaxo was already working on Flolan, and didn't think it was worth developing two pharmaceutical agents for an orphan disease that only affects a few thousand Americans, and possibly two hundred thousand people worldwide. They shelved this other substance and shifted to Flolan, which would obtain FDA approval in 1995.

Martine immediately latched on to this molecule. Crow cautioned her that it was just some chemical in the form of a powder that they had tried in rats. They had only published one article on it, filled with negative data. It was sitting on some shelf in the basement of a Glaxo facility gathering dust. Glaxo would never do anything with it. There just wasn't enough of a market there, and it would compete with their own drug anyways. Martine didn't listen to this part of the conversation. There was a drug. There was a chance for a cure. That was all she needed to know.

Martine called every Glaxo representative she could find. Once it became clear to her that Glaxo would not make any effort to develop it, she proposed the plan that her foundation would do it. She would hire experts to perform all the research. Glaxo declined, explaining to Martine that foundations aren't set up to develop and shepherd a drug through the FDA approval process. Martine kept pushing, and finally a Glaxo executive told her if she really wanted to do this, which in their opinion was foolhardy, Martine would need to form a pharmaceutical company and convince fifteen Glaxo executives to sign off on the deal. She would need to pay Glaxo for the patent rights, and if the drug ever came to fruition, pay a percentage of the profit to Glaxo in perpetuity. They were convinced that was the last they would see of Martine Rothblatt.

Perhaps any reasonable person would have gotten the message. But Martine had been disregarding the naysayers her entire life. She had already conquered space and gender. How hard could it be to start a pharmaceutical company? Martine sold the majority of her remaining equity in Sirius and other satellite firms, and invested $3 million into her new pharma company, which she would call United Therapeutics. She then approached many of her previous investors and friends with deep pockets. She approached banks, venture capital firms, billionaires—all the people who had believed in her before, and who had made a lot of money off this belief. This time, Martine was approaching these investors as a woman for the first time. Rather than deter anyone, Martine's transition was seen as a positive. "It burnished her status as self-made, a pioneer."[16] Martine quickly raised all the money she needed.

Martine made herself the CEO, drawing a salary of $75,000 per year. She brought on Crow as the president and chief operating officer. She reached out to prominent scientists around the world, forming an advisory board that included a Nobel Prize laureate and major figures in the pharmaceutical industry. She was in contact with executives at Glaxo daily, coaxing them to sign over this molecule. In a stroke of luck, the head of research at the company, a man named Bob Bell, happened to have a sister with PPH. He was moved by Martine's story and threw his support behind her. Slowly but surely, Martine obtained the necessary fifteen executive signatures to formalize the relationship, most likely to get her out of their hair.

Seven months after forming United Therapeutics, Martine obtained rights to the molecule. All Glaxo asked for was $25,000 and ten percent of any money she would make off it. They assumed the $25,000 was all they would ever see. Little did they know, given the return on investment, this would be the most lucrative deal Glaxo would ever make.

* * * * *

Martine's leadership style includes setting specific goals that will have meaning for her employees, her customers, and the world. She sets daily goals, attainable yearly goals, and more aspirational five-year goals. Her yearly goal when she started United Therapeutics was to identify a drug for PPH that could be administered without continuous injection. Her five-year goal was to have it on the market. Beyond that, she wanted it either inhaled or in a pill form.

Martine was admittedly surprised when she first laid eyes on this molecule that she had worked so hard to obtain. It was a small amount of powder that arrived in a little plastic sandwich bag. She must have felt a bit like a neighborhood drug dealer.

The scientists at Glaxo were sure she would fail. They knew the molecule had a very short half-life, was not in a form that could be given to a patient, and would cost too much to make it worthwhile for such a small market.

Martine knew they were wrong. She looked at patient adoption of her drug much like she looked at the growth of a subscription model for satellite radio—another concept that everyone told her would fail. She would pick up patients slowly but surely. As more patients were diagnosed with the disease and needed the drug, her profits would grow, and at the same time, she wouldn't lose her early "subscribers," who would likely need the drug for their lifetime. She also knew that the only competition in this market was Glaxo. No other pharma company was interested in anything related to PPH.

This fit with Martine's major philosophy she still holds today about start-ing a business in a new market, a philosophy she learned from Jack Welch when she was at UCLA business school. "Identify the corridors of indiffer-ence and run like hell down them. Find a market area that is ignored, has an unmet need. It's better to be a big fish in a small pond then a small fish in a big pond. If you can't be number one or number two, don't try."[17] Martine knew she could be at least number two in this market. She was confident she could become number one if she could make her drug inhalable.

The next few years were challenging. Progress was slow, but Martine kept things moving forward. She set her daily and weekly targets, with clear milestones. If the milestones weren't met, that particular avenue was shut down. She encouraged input and lively discussion about ideas, but herself remained the final word, the referee, the decision maker. She was the rare CEO that is both a visionary and a daily manager.

By three years, Martine took United Therapeutics public. By six years, the FDA approved United Therapeutics's first version of this molecule as an actual drug, under the trade name Remodulin. It wasn't an inhaled version (that avenue had to be temporarily diverted), but was approved for injection under the skin; it was much simpler and better tolerated than the rival Flolan.

With one approved drug under its belt, United Therapeutics began to expand its work into other orphan diseases, other corridors where United Therapeutics could quickly become number one or two. Martine's original five-year goal of a pill was becoming a reality, as trials for both inhaled and ingested versions of Remodulin were under way. Jenesis herself was thriving, growing into a healthy young woman who remained responsive to calcium channel blockers. She hadn't yet needed to take Remodulin or Flolan, but Martine still worried about her. No one knew how long Jenesis would stay responsive to her current treatment regimen, or what the possible long-term effects of the high blood pressure would have on her lungs and their longevity.

What if Jenny's lungs failed, what would happen then? Was it possible she would need them replaced someday? The need for a lung transplant had been on Martine's radar screen from the day Jenesis was given her diagnosis of PPH. Martine knew mastery of the transplant market wouldn't fit into a five-year plan. The complexity of the field was too high, and the science wasn't there yet to make a major innovation. But from those earliest days of her re-education, when she was reading everything that was known about lung physiology and treatment of lung disease, she was also exploring transplantation. She grasped the challenges of the field, the details that lead to poor outcomes for lung transplants, and the biggest barrier that everyone in transplant faced. There just weren't enough organs. Even in those early days of her re-education, Martine became aware that like every other problem she had encountered, there was a solution. The timing just had to be right.

* * * * *

Joe Tector was nineteen years old when he figured out what he wanted to do with the rest of his life. It was an October morning in 1984, and Len Bailey had just transplanted a baboon heart into Baby Fae. "I remember where I was when the news broke," he says. "At that moment I knew exactly what I wanted to do with my life."[18] Tector keeps a framed picture of Baby Fae in his office, inscribed to him by Leonard Bailey himself. It sits among pictures of Tector's children; if you didn't look that carefully, you might think Fae was one of them.

It wasn't that Tector just wanted to be a surgeon—he already knew that. It wasn't just that he wanted to be the best surgeon in the world—he already knew that as well. Tector wanted to do something that no one had ever done before. Xenotransplantation would fit that bill. Tector was smart enough to know that Baby Fae was just the start, that it would be decades before xenotransplantation could actually work. That was exactly the kind of life-mission Tector was looking for. It wasn't enough for Tector, the chronic underachiever as a boy growing up in Milwaukee, to defy the odds and become a surgeon. His father was already a virtuoso cardiac surgeon who performed more than fourteen thousand open-heart surgeries in his career, saving thousands of people with his skills and innovation. By the time Tector was in high school, he had watched his dad perform more complex cardiac surgeries than most surgery residents had seen. By the time Tector got to college at Indiana, he figured he could probably perform a cardiac bypass on his own.

When you sit with Tector and talk to him about his own life, it isn't long before he launches into a story about his dad, with a smile creeping across his face and a glint entering his eyes. By the end of the story, he is usually shaking his head in disbelief about whatever complex operation his dad had perfected.

There was the time when Tector and his brother Matt had gone with their dad to a Brewers game. He remembers sitting in the front seat of the car playing with some sort of strange toy—it looked like a big, curved straw. He couldn't understand why his dad had it in his car, and when he asked, his dad laughed and told him to put it back in the glove compartment. A couple of hours later, about six innings into the game, Tector heard his dad's name over the loudspeaker. "Dr. Cy Tector, can you please call your office?" The two boys walked with their dad to an office in the Milwaukee County Stadium, and after a short conversation, Cy told his sons they had to go. He had an emergency. Just a few hours later, Cy would be placing that funny looking tube Tector was playing with into a patient's chest, utilizing a novel technique to replace the aortic arch off the heart. It was one of the first times this was ever accomplished.

Or there was the time when Tector flew out to Utah with his dad when he was going to learn how to implant the Jarvik mechanical heart. There was an animal lab set up, and Cy would be implanting the heart into an anesthetized cow. After a brief demonstration by the inventors, Tector watched while his dad scrubbed in and removed the heart from his cow. Then he took the Jarvik heart and started trimming the cuff that was part of the mechanical heart. Jarvik ran over horrified, but Cy told him to relax, he thought he could improve it. Tector and Jarvik watched in awe as Cy rapidly sewed in this modified mechanical heart with such speed and grace. It fit so naturally that Jarvik himself explanted the modified heart to copy it for his next version.

Back in 1984, a few months before Len Bailey performed his inspirational xeno-heart transplant in October, Tector watched his dad perform his first heart transplant. It was like watching magic, or witchcraft. When he saw how beautifully his dad sewed that heart in place, and when it began beating—slowly at first, and then faster, more coordinated, until it was actually supporting the patient—Tector was mesmerized. He watched his dad perform countless more transplants over the next few years, and he never lost that feeling of awe. When Len Bailey did that baboon transplant, and his dad reacted with admiration, respect, and wonder at the courage of Bailey, he was intrigued. When his dad said it could never work, Tector had found his calling. He never looked back.

After college at Indiana University, Tector decided to spend the summer in a transplant research lab. It was the summer of 1988, and he found himself in Pittsburgh, where he met the man who would become the second most influential person in his life—Dr. Tom Starzl. It wasn't by chance that Tector ended up there. He wanted to work for the legendary transplant surgeon. At first he found himself ignored, which didn't surprise him. What could a recent college graduate possibly have to offer Starzl, the busiest and most prominent transplant surgeon in the world?

But one day, a senior researcher in the lab asked Tector to move all the equipment and papers out of an adjoining lab, because Starzl needed more space. After a few hours of work, Tector had the place nearly empty. As he was moving the last traces of someone's equipment into an abandoned lab closet, Tector heard the thundering voice of another surgeon he had seen around. "What the hell are you doing? Who the hell told you to move my stuff out of my damn lab?!" Tector recognized the name on this guy's badge—it was the same as the name on the label of the centrifuge he had moved into the shared equipment closet. "Sorry sir, I was told to help you move out of the lab." "Who the hell told you to do that?!" screamed this now red-faced man with the white hair and barrel-shaped chest. Tector wouldn't answer him. He just stood there quietly, keeping his eyes laser-focused on this man's gaze. Eventually the surgeon walked off in a huff, and Tector heard laughing from next door. When Starzl caught wind of it, he was entertained. When he heard Tector stayed silent under the inquisition by this cantankerous surgeon, Starzl was impressed. Maybe this student was worth something.

Tector spent the next four months in Starzl's presence every possible second. Starzl didn't sleep, never left work. Same with Tector. He would accompany Starzl on organ procurements and stand in the operating room watching him operate. His style was different than Cy's, who was always calm and soft-spoken, but they were both master surgeons. Tector was there when Starzl's team was experimenting with FK506, the drug that displaced cyclosporine as the mainstay of immunosuppression for organ transplantation to this day. Tector read everything that Starzl had written—which was a lot, as Starzl has more than 2,200 manuscripts to his name. Tector witnessed the power that Starzl yielded, but he also saw the other side of it. He saw how Starzl faced attacks from every angle. Starzl was always pushing the limits, taking on new risks, whether it be sicker and sicker patients that no one else would consider for transplant, trialing new medications like FK506, or even transplanting primate organs into humans, something he would do just a few years after Tector's time there. As Starzl liked to say, "I've always found that the best way to get a job done is to get the job done before anyone realizes what you are up to."[19] Tector watched people go after Starzl, both in public and in private. He understood the struggle of being a pioneer. Tector saw Starzl rejoice in his many victories, but also witnessed Starzl's exhaustion, how much it all weighed on him. Tector and Starzl talked about his plan to devote his career to making xenotransplantation a reality. Starzl warned Tector that it wasn't going to be easy. The doubters will be everywhere. He explained that if he really wanted to innovate at that level, he would suffer greatly. Starzl gave Tector one piece of advice: "Keep reading Winston Churchill. It will all become clear."

After medical school at St. Louis University, Tector performed his surgical residency at McGill University in Montreal. As an intern on the cardiac service, Tector realized he was more experienced in heart surgery than the new fellows. Tector, the intern, had some tricks to teach the fully trained cardiac surgeons. How would that go over? That wasn't something that worried Tector. He was a born alpha male. As he once told me, "I am Alfred Joseph Tector the third. My father did more cardiac bypasses than anyone in the world. I never saw that as a pressure." When the surgeons were coming off bypass in one of the first cases he scrubbed on, he noticed the fellow reaching for the defibrillator to shock the heart back to life. Tector mentioned that they didn't need to use the electricity, that his dad had taught him how to coax the heart back to life with his hands. The surgeons were surprised. They laughed. Sure, Joe, let's see what you can do. So Tector reached over and performed his dad's patented massage-and-flick move. Sure enough, the heart kicked into gear.

A few months later, Tector was scrubbed on a complex valve replacement. After completing the valve, the surgeon was unable to get the patient off bypass. Every time he tried to reduce the flow of the bypass pump, the heart struggled, unable to generate enough circulation to keep the patient alive. "Joe, your dad teach you any ideas here?" the lead surgeon asked him, half-jokingly? "Well, actually, Dad said any time you can't come off bypass after an aortic valve, you should bypass the right coronary. He said you probably narrowed its takeoff with the ring of the valve." It worked.

By the time Tector was a senior resident in Montreal, he was practically running the transplant service there. He was taking organ procurement call even while he was on other clinical services. He went on the majority of the procurements. He scrubbed on every liver transplant. Tector absolutely loved his time on the transplant service in Montreal. It was there that he proved to himself he could master transplantation, and it was there that he knew he had found his calling. He still considers his time there a life-altering experience and is deeply appreciative for the opportunities he was given.

While I had always assumed Tector was a natural surgeon, born with a gift for seeing the planes and always knowing where to focus during an operation, he recently told me that is not the case. When he first observed his father in surgery, he wondered to himself whether he would ever be able to do it. "Surgical skill is something that is a learned skill for everyone, that is one thing my father instilled into my head. I was terrible when I started, and it took a while before I could understand where to go from a tissue plane perspective. Clearly I was able to overcome this limitation and become proficient." So Tector wasn't born with the innate skill of surgery. But he was born with the traits of perseverance, endurance, and passion. He also had a strong desire not to embarrass himself, or his father. His confidence in surgery came from his intense work ethic, which solidified during his time in Montreal.

As Tector's experience grew, he started pushing the limits for what the Montreal program could take on. He remembers a young patient who presented in acute liver failure. Tector knew of the reports utilizing pig livers to keep patients alive until a human liver could become available. He convinced his attendings to let him give it a try. He found himself a pig and brought it to the animal lab. He removed the liver, brought it up to the ICU in a sterile basin, and attached it to the patient's blood vessels through large cannulas. Tector sat by his bedside for two days, going through three pig livers, until a human organ became available. The surgery was a success.

When Tector called his dad to tell him what he had just done, how he had saved his first patient with a xenotransplant of sorts, his dad answered the phone in a whisper. "What's that, Joe? Oh, that's great. Hey listen, I can't really talk now." Tector asked him why he was whispering. His dad told him to turn on the televsion. He was doing a national interview describing his tenth Jarvik artificial heart implant.

* * * * *

Tector's next stop was Miami, where he would conduct his transplant surgery fellowship. Two final years of training focused entirely on the care of transplant patients. There was something fitting about Tector being at Miami—it was where Starzl himself completed his own training in surgery. Tector performed transplants day and night. He honed his skills in this final chapter of his training, preparing to go out in the world and build something. He was becoming the type of surgeon he wanted to be—fast, confident, comfortable taking on the biggest cases he could find. But he also developed some enemies there and had his first taste of conflict. In residency, he always felt supported, loved, a total team player. In fellowship, he found that certain faculty were in his corner, but others fit into a category he might call "enemies"—people who wanted him to fail. This was the first time Tector noted he might be a polarizing figure.

Tector took his first job out of training at the Indiana School of Medicine in Indianapolis, where he had gone to college a decade before. At the time, Indiana had a middling transplant program surrounded by a bunch of bigger powerhouse programs in the Midwest. Tector was planning to change that. He signed on to Indiana with a small paycheck, but an opportunity to grow their liver transplant volume. Tector didn't care about money, at least money for his own personal use. He wanted to build something, and he saw an opportunity there. He knew they were underperforming, and he had the skills and confidence to change that.

In Tector's first year at Indiana, he performed 101 liver transplants himself. He was working day and night, in the Starzl model. He would fly out and get the organ from the donor, then fly back and sew it in. He honed his speed and skill, always thinking about how his father Cy would operate. Tector wanted his own cases to be like symphonies, and he pushed himself to move faster and further. His outcomes were excellent. He was blowing up the resources at Indiana—they didn't have enough ICU beds, nurses, operating rooms to sustain Tector's trajectory. But he didn't care. He kept listing sick patients, the sicker the better. He kept accepting liver offers, transplanting them day and night.

Within two years, Tector was the head of the liver transplant service. His was the busiest service in the hospital, and it was bringing in more money than any other service in the hospital system. But he wasn't satisfied. He decided he would add a multivisceral program to their repertoire. This rare operation builds on a liver transplant, for patients who lack adequate intestines and have to take their nutrition intravenously. In the operation, first successfully performed by Starzl in 1987, surgeons transplant the liver, stomach, pancreas, and small bowel all at once—essentially an abdomen transplant. Tector performed his first multivisceral transplant in 2003, and by 2009 had done a hundred. Tector tells the story of his first, how smoothly it went and how proud he was. That evening, despite having been awake for the better part of two days, Tector called home before he went to bed. He reached his mother Joy, a retired operating room nurse. Cy was the famous heart surgeon, but it was Joy who was in charge of their family life. As much as Joy loved her family, and her family loved her, she was fiercely loyal to Cy. No one, even her own children, could compete with him. As Tector excitedly reported that he had just transplanted a liver, stomach, pancreas, and small bowel into a small child, he already knew what her response would be. "Yeah, well did you hear what your father just did?"

But Tector knew his parents were on vacation at their lake house, so he couldn't imagine that he had just done some sort of novel heart operation. Instead, Cy saw smoke coming out of a neighbor's house. He ran right to the door, where he put his hand on it and felt heat. In he ran, and a few minutes later came running out with one of their neighbors slumped over his shoulders! As if that wasn't enough, he ran back in and pulled out her husband.

Tector rolled his eyes and laughed as he recounted this story. "Oh, Joy" he said with a chuckle. He loved his mother, who had just died six months earlier. She was the rock of the family. But for all Tector's accomplishments, he could never impress her.

* * * * *

In 2006, Tector began negotiating with the leadership at Indiana University Hospital to create a proposed Indiana University Health Transplant Institute. This would be separate from any other department, so he would report directly to the leadership of the health system. In his proposal, Tector would control his own funds, with the ability to use clinical dollars generated by the institute to fund education, clinical hires, and research. In early 2007, Tector became chief medical officer at the Indiana University Health Transplant Institute, medical director of organ transplantation, and a member of the Board of Trustees at Indiana University. He would become its chairperson a few years later.

So finally, in 2007, Tector was ready to dig in. He was well acquainted with the advances in xenotransplantation since the generation of the Alpha Gal knockout. He was also aware that they were limited. He knew the data out of the Sachs lab using their knockout in transplants, with and without the thymus, and their continued pursuit of transplant tolerance. He knew the results in Pittsburgh using the Ayares pigs, with Cooper now running the preclinical models transplanting organs into primates. He knew that Ayares had added a complement regulatory protein to his Alpha Gal knockout, with limited improvement in graft survival.

He wasn't exactly sure what novel angle he could add to the work being done, but he figured he would start transplanting some of these transgenic pigs and see what happened. He reached out to Ayares and Sachs to ask for some knockout pigs that he could use. Unfortunately, they said no. Sachs just didn't have enough animals at the time. Ayares similarly was limited, with Cooper transplanting the majority of his pigs. He told Tector he couldn't help him either.

Tector did a few experiments using outbred pigs, perfusing some human blood through them and looking at the effect on platelets. But he realized rather quickly that this would never get him anywhere. He needed a reliable source of transgenic pigs. Tector thought about contracting his gene editing and cloning to an outside facility, like the one Sachs had used in Missouri. Homologous recombination seemed like a tricky business, and what did Tector know about cloning? But the more he thought about it, the more he realized he needed to make his own pigs. He didn't want to be beholden to anyone to have animals to work with.

But there was something more compelling. Tector figured there were loads of surgeons out there who could transplant pig organs into primates, and eventually into people. In order to move the needle on this perplexing field, he would need to embrace the generation of the pigs themselves. Successful xenotransplantation from pigs was going to require designer animals. Tector had a long-term vision, and that vision required "making" the organs that would transform the field of medicine.

Tector understood that he needed to make a pig that could be transplanted across this chasm protected by natural antibodes against Gal and likely some other targets. He could also see that Ayares, Sachs, and others in the xeno community were already focusing on more complex gene edits, knocking out receptors that would stimulate the human immune cells and cause rejection, or knocking in proteins that would regulate the immune response after transplant. Tector had a different strategy in mind. He surmised that staying simple and relying on what we already knew about allotransplantation (human to human transplantation) would be the most realistic route. A simple edit like knocking out Alpha Gal might be enough for some people, whose immune systems were naïve and responded well to available immunosuppression, but other patients may need a second knockout, or a third. He wanted to go stepwise, to keep it simple, and then widen the net and help more patients. He worried that complex edits, particularly those that added new genes, might have unpredictable effects on the organs themselves. And he knew, even in 2007, that getting a pig with numerous edits in its genome approved by the FDA would be difficult.

So Tector would start making pigs. He would develop mastery of each step of the process in house, either on his own or by hiring an expert. Step one would be learning how to clone a pig. It had been less than a decade since Dolly was cloned with nuclear transfer, and half that since the very first pig was successfully cloned. There were only a handful of labs in the world that could do this in the first decade of the 2000s, only one of which was focused solely on transplant—Ayares's lab in Virginia. As Ayares has admitted, he's not a transplant surgeon; he's a geneticist. He relies on immunologists and transplant surgeons to tell him which genes to go after. Tector's lab would be the first fully functional, vertically integrated xenotransplantation program.

The first hire Tector made would be one of the most fortuitous moves of his xeno career. He recruited Jose Estrada, a junior researcher from North Carolina who was part of a lab performing somatic cell nuclear transfer at a veterinary school in North Carolina. Cloning is a tricky, fickle business and requires a combination of innate skill, practice, patience, and persistence beyond any reasonable expectation. Estrada had all of the innate characteristics, and just needed more practice. That he got in Tector's lab. They would run experiments day and night. Tector would show up for many of them, even though he was still the surgeon of record for almost every liver and small bowel transplant performed at Indiana. He wanted to understand every aspect of the process, and he knew he couldn't do that by just hearing about what was done. He had to be part of it.

The cloning would be worthless without mastering the gene editing. Although Tector was confident he and Estrada could master the cloning, he felt more intimidated by the techniques of gene editing. He knew a bit about homologous recombination, and how inefficient and frustrating a process it was. The idea that it might take a year to generate a transgenic mouse, that the odds of achieving the modification you were interested in was something like one in a million, was a major turnoff to Tector. But he also had read that something new was on the horizon—a technique known as "zinc finger nucleases."

It hadn't yet been used to make a transgenic animal but was successful at targeting and editing genes in cells. Tector didn't know anything about zinc, and figured he was too busy to figure it out on his own. While Tector focused on the nuclear transfer, he hired a PhD with experience in gene editing. After a few months, this new scientist was showing off his gene therapy success in pig fibroblasts—a somatic connective tissue cell that was typically used to generate the Alpha Gal knockout pigs. It wouldn't be long before Tector's group would be able to make a knockout pig themselves.

But he recognized a problem—this gene editor was good at working with cells, but less good at working with people. Initially Tector didn't really mind that. He himself could get frustrated by social interactions and was way more interested in results than small talk. If he wanted a friend, he could get a dog. (These days, Tector has a Chihuahua. He looks ridiculous with it—such an imposing, intense guy with such a little dog.) But one day this gene editor came into Tector's office and told him he needed to get rid of most everyone else in the lab. They were annoying him and he couldn't work with them. Tector hesitated; he knew he couldn't fire everyone in the lab. But could he get by without this scientist? As Tector thought about it, he came to a quick conclusion. He would learn gene editing himself. How hard could it be? "I have a solution to our problems. You're fired."

Tector set his sights on becoming the best gene editor in the world. He hit the books, reading everything he could about gene editing, starting with the work of James D. Watson and Francis Crick, re-reading all of Oliver Smithies's papers, slowly making his way to modern editing techniques. When Tector reads a paper, he doesn't just get the general gist of it—he inhales it, he studies it, looks up all the references. (He essentially memorizes it. I have had numerous conversations with Tector where he starts quoting from random scientific papers that he read years ago.) If something doesn't make sense to him, he reaches out to the author or other experts in the field. Then he tries the experiments himself.

Once Tector understood homologous recombination, he decided it was time to move on to zinc finger nucleases. He discovered Eric Lander, the brilliant Harvard molecular biologist/geneticist who founded the Broad Institute and was one of the key figures in the Human Genome Project (HGP). Lander had recorded a number of lectures and courses on genes and genetic engineering. Tector likes to say that he attended night school at iTunes University. He would "attend" lectures in the middle of the night, in between cases or before meetings. Tector realized that with zinc fingers, he could finally start making the pigs he had been dreaming about.

* * * * *

So what is a zinc finger nuclease?[20] In short, another example of humans borrowing a process seen in nature to accomplish something spectacular. In 1985, a British scientist named Aaron Klug was investigating how certain genes in the DNA were suddenly transcribed to form a protein. He was studying a protein isolated from the xenopus (a type of frog) that had properties that allowed it to bind to specific nucleic acid sequences in DNA. This protein had interesting and unusual characteristics. It consisted of a string of specific base pairs held into a folded conformation by one or more zinc ions, which reliably included a finger-like structure that would protrude out and bind to specific DNA. Klug recognized that binding of this finger-like protein to specific spots in the DNA would serve as a signal to turn on the transcription of a gene (earning the name "transcription factor"). Klug found he could link a few zinc fingers together to specify exactly where on the genome they would bind. Each zinc finger would bind three base pairs of DNA, so by linking two or three zinc fingers together, he could design them to bind a stretch of DNA nine base pairs long, increasing the specificity.[21]

In 1996, a team at Johns Hopkins University in Baltimore fused a zinc finger protein, by now characterized according to what specific DNA it would bind, to an enzyme that acts like a scissors and cuts both strands of DNA.[22] This enzyme, called an endonuclease, was discovered in the 1960s as a tool bacteria use for their own protection against invading viruses, but it wasn't until the generation of this fusion protein that the potential to harness this effect for gene editing was realized. They now had a strategy to design a tandem of specific zinc fingers that would bind a specific gene or length of DNA hidden within the three billion base pairs packed into a human or animal cell, and then the endonuclease would cut that DNA out, allowing an edit.

Various groups spent the next decade characterizing what happens when a double-stranded DNA around a gene of interest is cut. Cells have natural repair processes built in to repair breaks in DNA, as these occur naturally throughout the life of an organism. The simplest repair involves the DNA just joining back together right at the site of the double-stranded break, a process termed nonhomologous end joining. In other words, the DNA just rejoins with the cut-out piece now gone, sometimes called a "frame-shift." This results in a simple knockout of a specified gene. The second process of repair is termed homology-directed repair, which is the same process described in homologous recombination. Scientists figured out that if they injected a specific DNA template encoding a gene they were interested in adding, flanked by "arms" of base pairs that match the DNA at the double stranded cut, the gene would be inserted by the mechanism of homologous recombination. Although this technique was still painstaking and time-consuming, with many failures and off target effects, it is between ten thousand and one hundred thousand times more efficient than homologous recombination alone. By the 2010s, labs were becoming efficient at designing highly specific zinc fingers, and gene-editing companies were formed that would allow researchers to order designer zinc fingers specifying particular genes to target for removal or insertion.

* * * * *

Tector learned this and so much more by reading, listening to online lectures, and trying various techniques out in the lab. Each time he failed to edit a gene, he would reach out to the authors of the various papers and run through the techniques with them. Eventually he got the knack for it. Name a gene, and Tector could design zinc fingers for it and knock it out in a pig cell.

Tector had set up his entire clinical operation to support his ability to achieve his research goals. When he accepted a liver for transplant, he would take a team approach to its implantation. One of his junior partners would go out and procure the organ, while another began removing the liver from the recipient. When they were ready for him, Tector would come from the lab and sew it in. Once the liver was sewn in and re-perfused (filled with blood), Tector would return to the lab while his partners would close up the patient and get ready for the next transplant. The massive transplant institute was generating so much money that Tector was able to support his research with excess clinical dollars, in addition to the many government grants they were able to obtain.

Tector's lab made its first small advance in 2011, when it succeeded in isolating fetal liver cells from Alpha Gal knockout pigs and placed them in culture, and were able to keep them alive for months. They then were able to take these cells out of culture and perform nuclear transfer, generating Alpha Gal knockout clones from these cells.[23] Then, a year later, Tector's group mastered gene editing using zinc finger nucleases and used these gene-edited cells to clone a pig. They made their first gene-edited Alpha Gal knockout by early 2012.[24]

Next, Tector took cells from his Alpha Gal knockouts and mixed them with human serum, and then analyzed the antibody that still bound to the cells. He employed advanced techniques to delineate these antigens, and then identified what genes were responsible for these proteins. He then scoured the literature for what was known about antibodies, proteins, genes—anything that was present in pigs but no longer expressed in humans, lost by the discriminatory process of evolution. Tector stumbled on a particular enzyme (CMAH) and a carbohydrate it generated (Neu5Gc) that were found to be lacking in humans and present in horses, and which were responsible for the serum sickness response seen in humans exposed to antiserum against tetanus and diphtheria generated in horses. Roughly two million years ago, a mutation in the CMAH gene got fixed into the human lineage, which made it impossible for humans to generate the Neu5Gc carbohydrate. This mutation did not occur in other primates or any other mammal, all of whom still generate this carbohydrate. Humans develop anti-Neu5Gc antibodies early in life, both from exposure to this carbohydrate in diet (including the meat and milk from animals that express this antigen) and exposure to gut bacteria that, similar to Alpha Gal, express this carbohydrate in their cell wall.

Tector understood that all humans begin expressing this antibody shortly after birth, and virtually all other mammals express the target this antibody binds to on their cell surfaces. This was obviously a barrier to successful transplantation of animal organs to humans. CMAH would be the next gene Tector would knock out. He would simply be accelerating millions of years of evolution one gene at a time.

First, Tector's team designed a zinc finger nuclease that could bind and cleave the CMAH gene, and performed gene therapy on porcine liver-derived cells to knock this enzyme and Alpha Gal out. Once they identified cells that had both of these genes knocked out, somatic cell nuclear transfer was performed using mature enucleated oocytes. These oocytes were then transferred into pigs on their first day of estrus. They transferred roughly a hundred embryos into each of two surrogate pigs. One of the surrogates failed to generate any fetuses, but the second had five. These were harvested at thirty days, and the fetuses were tested to ensure they were truly double knockouts. After successfully confirming this, fetal fibroblasts were harvested and four surrogates received more than a hundred embryos each using these fetal fibroblasts in the nuclear transfer process. Only one of these surrogates became successfully pregnant, but from that pig, four double knockout pigs were born.[25]

The process was tedious and challenging, but in the end, it took seven months to generate four double knockout pigs. Tector tested human blood against cells from these pigs and found a dramatic reduction in antibody response compared to the Alpha Gal knockout.[26] Tector understood that the CMAH knockout would have little effect on binding when he mixed cells from these knockout pigs with primate blood, as primates had the CMAH gene (unlike humans) and hence had no antibodies against the carbohydrate made by this gene. But he was surprised to find that in fact the antibodies in baboon blood bound stronger to cells from these pigs.[27] It turns out knocking out this gene led to the generation of a novel antigen that primates have antibodies against. Tector recognized this would make things more challenging in the pre-clinical animal models, since it would make the outcomes worse in pig-to-primate transplant. But he knew that when it came to human xenotransplantation, it would reduce the relevant natural antibody in humans that would bind to the pig organs.

Tector was ever more convinced that success would be based on minimizing the targets of pre-formed antibody with genetic modifications in the pigs, and then using immunosuppression to address the T cell responses. In one rather compelling set of experiments, he compared the human antibody response to his double knockout (Alpha Gal and CMAH) pigs to the human response to chimpanzee cells. Much to Tector's surprise, his double knockout pigs caused a much smaller antibody response than chimpanzee cells![28] In other words, the human serum attacked the chimpanzee cells more than the pig cells. Tector wasn't satisfied yet. While generating these novel pigs, he was simultaneously testing hundreds of human serum samples against cells from his knockout pigs. He found that at least a quarter of them had completely negative crossmatches, with no evidence of antibody against modified pig cells. A similar amount had low-level antibodies, which would probably be manageable by immunosuppressive strategies already in use in humans.

But Tector wanted to do better. He continued to scour the literature, and test human and primate samples against pig cells to identify more carbohydrates to knock out.

* * * * *

One early morning at 2:00 a.m., in the first week of March of 2013, Tector had finished sewing in a liver and had a few hours before the next one. He was casually flipping through the February 15 issue of *Science*, when he noticed two articles that ran back to back on a new system for gene editing. The title of the first was "Multiplex genome engineering using CRISPR/Cas systems."[29] The second was "RNA-guided human genome engineering via Cas9."[30] They both came out of Boston, out of the Broad Institute of MIT and Harvard started by his scientific idol, Eric Lander. As he dove into the first article, he knew his world was about to change. This was his first time reading about the CRISPR-Cas system for gene editing, and he was enthralled. Tector read and re-read the methods section, picturing every step of the process, committing it to memory. It was so simple, so beautiful . . . so obvious.

So what is CRISPR-Cas9?[31] It is a gene editing system that is—like everything cool in scientific discovery—borrowed from another organism that already uses it. Bacteria utilize a version of this system in their primitive immune system. When bacteria get infected by a virus, they insert pieces of the viral DNA in their own genome, in specific patterns or clusters (termed "clustered regularly interspaced short palindromic repeats," or CRISPRs). These strange palindromic repeats were identified as early as the late 1980s, and characterized well enough to be given the name "CRISPR" in 2001. It was later discovered that if these bacteria are then invaded by the same virus, they generate RNA fragments from the CRISPR repeats that attach to the viral DNA, and then release the Cas9 endonuclease that cuts the virus apart, as a primitive memory response to the virus. In other words, the bacteria keep a blueprint of the virus the first time it is encountered, and then when they get re-infected, they use this blueprint to generate a targeted memory response that can cleave the virus.

Researchers including Jennifer Doudna, Emmanuelle Charpentier, George Church, and Feng Zhang figured out how to adapt this system for gene editing.[32] They showed that by generating a short segment of RNA with a guide sequence specific for a particular gene in the genome (the CRISPR), and attaching it to the Cas9 enzyme, it could be inserted into the cell, causing a cut in the DNA at that specific spot. Then, similar to the case with zinc finger nucleases, the DNA either repairs itself primarily, or the DNA encoding a new gene is injected and then inserted into the cut segment. This was a major advance from zinc finger nucleases, as the RNA targeting sequences are easy to design, there are fewer off target effects, and multiple genes can be targeted at once.

At the bottom of the first page, Tector saw the email for correspondences to the senior author, Feng Zhang. Tector immediately wrote a note to Dr. Zhang, explaining his interest in this new system. He asked Zhang where he might find the reagents to try this himself, or if he could come see them use it in Boston.

A couple weeks later, Tector came down to his office from the OR at 10 a.m., after another all-night transplant-athon. He hadn't slept in two nights, but that didn't really bother him. When he sat at his desk, he saw a note from his assistant, letting him know that some guy from Harvard sent him a package. Tector ripped open the express mail envelope, and inside he found some vials on ice. Zhang had sent him plasmids for the Cas9 enzyme, CRISPR RNAs, and a methods sheet on how to proceed. Zhang's lab had put together a "do-it-yourself" CRISPR gene editing kit, with everything he would need to get started. Tector canceled all his meetings and ran straight down to the lab.

Once Tector had CRISPR-Cas9 up and running, he became a man on a mission looking for genes to edit. Each time he identified a new potential gene candidate that might encode a xeno-antigen, he would knock it out of pig cells and test the antibody response against human and primate serum. If it seemed interesting, he would go on and generate a knockout pig. He even perfected generating different knockout piglets in the same surrogate sow! He could thus have one sow birth a single Alpha Gal knockout, an Alpha Gal/CMAH knockout, and a triple knockout that included some other candidate gene.

After months of experimentation and literature review, Tector read about another gene (B4GALNT2) missing in five percent of the population that sometimes led to blood transfusion reactions due to natural antibodies. Five percent might not seem like a lot, but with the current kidney transplant waitlist at a hundred thousand people, five percent is still five thousand people. He called down to the lab and gave some directions.

In early 2015, Tector's group published its results with the triple knockout pig, a pig that had the Alpha Gal, CMAH, and B4GALNT2 genes knocked out of its genome, with the edits performed by CRISPR-Cas9 technology.[33] The animals were born healthy with normal organ function. When they tested human serum against cells from these pigs, they were excited to find that the majority of samples had major reductions in their antibody responses to the triple knockout. In fact, the majority of serum had no antibody at all. Rather than reducing the response in just five percent of samples, almost all of the samples seemed to harbor antibodies to the product of this gene. The data was compelling. Tector had his pig.

* * * * *

When Martine was first envisioning what United Therapeutics might accomplish, she set realistic goals for where the company might be in five and ten years. Within five years, she pictured a drug on the market that could compete with Flolan, something that didn't have to run through a continuous IV. Five years beyond that, she pictured having the drug in inhaled and ingested formats. These were ambitious goals considering where Martine was starting from. But they were also a bit banal for her. Martine was a world-changer, and simply running a pharmaceutical company was never going to be enough for her.

One innovation that was big enough for Martine, as transformational as sending satellites or people to space, caught her eye when she was spending a majority of her waking hours in her self-administered biological sciences curriculum. As she advanced through high school biology textbooks, college-level molecular biology, and medical school biochemistry and pharmacology, she found herself fascinated with the building blocks of genetics, from the structure of DNA to advances in gene sequencing and the developing techniques of gene editing. She was particularly intrigued by the size and scope of the Human Genome Project, officially launched in 1990. The goal of the project was simple—to sequence and identify all the base pairs that make up human DNA, and to map and sequence all of the genes in the human genome. This was the kind of landmark international collaboration that she could really get behind.

As she sat with her books in the medical library, Martine thought about her grandmother, whose life was saved when she received a pig valve that replaced her own failing heart valve. The valve her grandmother received was decellularized, essentially a mechanical replacement of the human valve that was failing before the rest of her body was. But she knew it represented something more than replacing her human valve with a man-made mechanical substitute. This was an example of borrowing from another species to replace a failing part. Martine grasped, as early as 1995, that if a pig valve could work in a human without any real modification, then the biochemistry of pig and human organs had to be more similar than dissimilar.

As Martine read about the work of David White and the hDAF pigs, and contemplated what the Human Genome Project was likely to accomplish over the next decade, she came to a conclusion. "I had known circa 1995 that I wanted to do Xeno to create an unlimited supply of organs."[34] Martine knew the timing wasn't ripe to jump into the xeno market; it wouldn't be an achievable five- or ten-year goal in 1995. But she also knew that it was much closer than critics understood. "I believed mechanistically that with the launched HGP that it was just a matter of time to identify and then edit away a handful of genes that caused rejection. How could function be so similar and biochemistry be completely dissimilar? Made no sense . . ."[35]

While Martine focused United Therapeutics on the business of bringing a drug to market, and concentrated her investor pitches on therapeutics for the underserved orphan disease PPH, she continued her own education in the discipline of xenotransplantation, including the science of genetics, the players in the field, and the barriers. It became clear to her in the mid-1990s that the barriers would not be the genetics or the immune response. She never believed it would be necessary to modify hundreds of genes in pigs to make them acceptable to humans. She predicted it would be about a dozen genes that need to be modified, and saw that technology as a decade or two away. She also recognized that some of the most brilliant scientists in the world—people like Craig Venter, George Church, and Francis Collins—were devoting every waking moment to understanding genes and how to modify them. Martine would read everything she could about these efforts, but eventually, when the timing was right, when she could fit it into a five- or ten-year plan with realistic milestones, she would recruit her own team of superstars to help craft the pigs that would become an unlimited source of spare parts in her quest to replace failing organs.

The challenge that Martine perceived, that she pictured herself having to address as the CEO of an eventual company providing GMO organs off the shelf for humans, was from a different scientific discipline. She would be the face of an organization that would need to justify the ethics of breeding pigs to serve as organ donors, modifying their genes to make them more "human-like," and transplanting these organs across species into immunosuppressed hosts. The potential of introducing a novel virus, bacteria, or parasite that could cause a global pandemic did not seem too farfetched.

Martine thought this might be the "corridor" where she could develop some unique expertise and authority. She decided to pursue an advanced degree in bioethics. So while Martine was the CEO of a startup biopharmaceutical company, had just published a book on her own gender transition, and was still collaborating with major satellite communications corporations, she began a PhD in bioethics at the University of London. Martine completed her PhD with a dissertation on the ethics of xenotransplantation in 2001, which was published in 2003 under the title *Your Life or Mine: How Geoethics Can Resolve the Conflict Between Private and Public Interests in Xenotransplantation.*[36] The thesis reads like a handbook for how to safely and ethically run a xenotransplantation organization. It discusses the ethics of using animals as donors for humans, complete with a comprehensive review of philosophical opinions on animal research and specifications on how to treat the animals from birth until their donation. It includes a wide-ranging discussion of the risks of PERV and other potential xeno-viruses. Specific follow-up protocols and testing regimens are included in the dissertation, delineated to the smallest detail. There is discussion about the finances of a company that might be involved in providing organs for transplantation, with a novel protocol on how companies might provide for populations across the world that might not have the logistic or financial resources to safely conduct trials or provide follow-up care for patients in need. The thesis also addresses potential regulatory requirements for conducting trials and administering a market for xeno, delineating an ethical and practical framework for how the FDA and other regulatory bodies might proceed in the future. This thesis was essentially a business plan for a future version of United Therapeutics.

Martine was poised to enter the xeno-business. She was just waiting for the right time, the right opportunity.

* * * * *

It was the end of 2010, and David Ayares was exhausted. The last seven years at Revivicor had been filled with progress and excitement—in addition to the Alpha Gal knockouts, Ayares had added a variety of "combo"-transgenic pigs to his company's repertoire, including incorporating different human complement inhibitors onto the Gal knockout. Cooper was performing the pig-to-primate transplants at Pittsburgh, and slowly but surely the graft survival was improving, with triple-figure survival more the norm than the exception. Ayares was particularly excited with a couple of collaborations that were thriving—one with a brilliant Pakistani-born scientist by the name of Muhammad Mohiuddin at the NIH in Washington, DC, and one with a heart and lung transplant surgeon named Robin Pierson at the University of Maryland. His success was not limited to solid organ transplantation. Researchers at Pittsburgh were also making progress in developing models of islet transplantation, the cells in the pancreas that generate insulin and are missing in patients with Type I Diabetes. Modified pig cells promised to provide an unlimited supply of these cells, which were so hard to procure from deceased human donors of other organs.

Yet despite all the progress, all the papers, all the government funding and brilliant researchers, Ayares found himself out of money once again. He had hoped in 2003—after scratching and clawing his way to a solvent company with guaranteed funding from a leading academic institution, a massive pharmaceutical company, and major venture fund—that his problems with money were over. He enjoyed being CEO of Revivicor when his job was to lead teams, think about what pigs to produce, initiate collaborations, and plan experiments. Fundraising, in his mind, was for the birds. But now, here he was at the end of 2010, with enough money left for two months of operations. Two months! After that, he wouldn't make payroll. He wouldn't even be able to pay his own salary. Even worse, he wouldn't have enough money to keep his beloved designer pigs alive.

Ayares had just hung up the phone with his managers at Pittsburgh's investment fund. They were pulling the plug on Revivicor. It was just too expensive, and while the University had an academic mission, the fund had a more capitalistic goal. Xeno just wasn't poised to bring in any money any time soon. Starzl, long retired from clinical duties at this point, couldn't convince them to keep floating this never-ending drag on their finances. Ayares had alerted Cooper, who was well versed in the chronic condition of dwindling finances. Such was the life of an academic. Ayares had a list of employees in front of him that he was planning to furlough.

When the phone rang, it took him a few beats to snap out of his doldrums. He wasn't really expecting any calls, and figured it could only be more bad news, someone wondering when his last check might clear.

Ayares remembers the call like it was yesterday, the blunt words spoken to him on a cold call imprinted in his brain forever. "I represent United Therapeutics. We are developing lung therapies. Martine Rothblatt is interested in your company. She wants to buy you." Ayares doesn't remember much else about the conversation, but he does admit that at the time, he didn't know who Martine Rothblatt was. After he hung up the phone, he googled her. His reaction to her story was that she was a true pioneer. And she was offering him a lifeline. He was going to grab it any way he could.

After Ayares hung up the phone with the United Therapeutics representative, one of the first calls he made was to Tom Starzl. Had he ever heard of Rothblatt, Ayares asked him? Of course he had. Apparently the world of pioneers was smaller than Ayares had realized. Martine had first reached out to Starzl when she was working on her PhD more than a decade before.

From her side, Martine knew exactly who Starzl was. She knew about his legendary exploits in the world of transplantation, and was aware of his forays into the discipline of xenotransplantation. One of Martine's tenets as a business leader was to amass expertise when taking on a new project. Her advisory boards were filled with Nobel Prize laureates, masters of industry, and academic superstars. Starzl agreed to serve on her PhD committee, and once that was completed, was a trusted advisor as she contemplated when she would make the jump into clinical xenotransplantation. They had earnest discussions after her 2008 induction into the American Philosophical Society, "the oldest learned society in the United States.'" Starzl had been inducted in 1999. It was then that he first told Martine about the company in Virginia that Pittsburgh was funding at his recommendation.

In 2010, Martine had decided it was time to get in to the xeno business. Gene editing had progressed beyond the days of homologous recombination, and it was possible to envision the generation of pigs with organs that could be accepted by humans. She reached out to Starzl to get his advice. It must have come as no surprise when he told her to call David Ayares.

* * * * *

Ayares spent the entire flight to Vermont going over his slide deck. He had given this investor talk hundreds of times over the last few years, but he was still nervous. This was his last chance to keep his company afloat. The thought of having to fire all those employees, uproot his family, and most horribly, to sacrifice all those pigs, made him sick to his stomach. He knew they had made so much progress, and was sure the reality of successful xenotransplantation was so close. He just needed to convince Martine, his white knight.

Ayares was led into a room in a beautiful Vermont house. He was wearing a suit and tie, had his notes before him, and his thirty slides ready to go. After what seemed like an eternity, the door opened and Martine ambled in, followed by two big labradoodles. She had a big smile and greeted him warmly. Ayares began his formal presentation, starting his talk with the early days of xeno, the discovery of Alpha Gal antibodies, his successful first knockout pig using homologous recombination. About halfway through his presentation Martine stopped him. "David, you can stop. I'm buying it. Let's go to lunch." Martine already knew everything about Revivicor. She knew all their accomplishments, their IP, their competitors, their employees, and their vision. She had been following their progress closely since 2008, with Starzl himself providing updates along the way. On their way to lunch, Martine called Starzl from her cellphone. "Tom, we are buying it!"

In July of 2011, United Therapeutics acquired Revivicor for a cool $7.6 million. Ayares would remain the CEO and would report directly to Martine. She was committed to spending the next decade deciding on genes to edit to provide an unlimited source of organs for human transplantation. Although Martine's passion, her drive, was to cure patients with end-stage lung disease, she was interested in a one-size-fits-all pig that could cure diseases of all organs. Martine had done the research, calculated the potential costs, and was confident this would be achievable. She predicted a decade was a realistic time frame for success. Ayares was finally able to take a deep breath. He would never need to worry about money again. Now he could focus on the science.

* * * * *

In 2012–2013, Jennifer Doudna and Emmanuelle Charpentier published a series of papers describing their success at harnessing CRISPR-Cas9.[37] They designed a simplified system to identify and cut a DNA target specified by guide RNA. They further demonstrated that they could alter the guide RNA and target any DNA sequence in bacteria. This was the culmination of the work of many researchers, including Feng Zhang at Harvard.[38] The new era of gene editing had begun. (Doudna and Charpentier would ultimately be awarded the 2020 Nobel Prize in chemistry, highlighting the importance of this discovery.)

Later that same year a Harvard geneticist named George Church published his description of using the CRISPR-Cas9 gene editing system for the first time in a human cell line.[39] Church had been at the forefront of genetic sequencing since its beginning, and is one of the initiators of the Human Genome Project in 1984. He had been involved in genome engineering and cloning since the 1980s. He or members of his lab at Harvard have co-founded more than fifty companies exploring technologies from anti-aging to personalized medicine to an effort to revive the woolly mammoth. His physical presence is as impressive as his academic achievements. He is tall and lanky, with a booming low voice and a big thick white beard. The person he most resembles is God. Church has definitely used this to his advantage.

He has a variable level of involvement in each of his companies, but his presence at investor meetings has never failed to raise big money from venture capital firms looking for the next transformative scientific advance. If you are a rich businessperson looking to change the world with your money, putting it into Church's next venture is never a bad strategy.

Church was well acquainted with xenotransplantation by this point. He remembered being fascinated by the Baby Fae case, although he was aware at that time that the science was not yet mature enough for the surgeon to have expected that effort to succeed. Church was a fan of optimists and risk-takers. But he was grounded in science first; he was not someone who would embark on a human or animal experiment that he hadn't thought through or didn't believe had a chance of succeeding. No such chance existed in 1984. But more recently, shortly after publication of his work using CRISPR in human cells, Church had been approached by Martine, Tector, and Sachs, each independently, to inquire if his lab would help the field with its "editing magic on dozens of target genes." As Church recounted to me, "It seemed like a very warm welcome." Church, having received more than ten thousand requests for his CRISPR plasmids by this point, recognized that the field of gene editing was exploding, and he immediately understood that xenotransplantation would open some novel avenues of experimentation for the lab.

Church had a student by the name of Luhan Yang, a brilliant and aggressive Chinese graduate student pursuing her PhD in his lab. Church had the utmost respect for Yang. He knew she came across as abrasive and overbearing to some, but he was confident that was a misread. She was just driven with a work ethic bordering on insane. Her direct approach and avoidance of small talk turned collaborators off, but she just didn't have enough time in the day to accomplish all the things she knew she was capable of. Church suggested to Luhan that she immerse herself in the growing literature on xenotransplantation, and identify some unique targets where they might apply their advanced gene editing techniques.

In 2014, Yang presented her proposal for a new xeno-related project. She had reviewed everything she could find related to the genes that had been targeted in xeno experiments. Most of the publications were in obscure journals, not *Nature*, *Science*, or *Cell*, where the Church lab commonly published. Their success was limited, but they had made a bit of progress, all while using relatively unsophisticated editing techniques. Most interesting to Yang was not the genes they had elected to modify, but instead the publications related to PERV, the porcine endogenous retrovirus that was present in virtually all pigs. From what Yang read, the discovery of PERV had essentially put a halt to any potential pig-to-human human xeno trials.

So when Yang proposed the idea to explore the pig genome and find all the places where PERV genes resided, and then cut them out with CRISPR-Cas9 gene editing, Church was intrigued. It did seem like an elegant way to solve a critical problem worth solving. Church didn't see PERV as some academic, clinically irrelevant issue that could be ignored. He read with concern all the papers and opinion pieces that minimized the PERV risk, predicting the chances of human infection were minimal, with the risk of a pandemic infinitesimal. He found the argument that humans have lived in close proximity to pigs for thousands of years to be unpersuasive. He was even more bothered by the opinion pieces that described the FDA as too risk adverse, being influenced by fears of the uneducated rather than driven by science. Church had a specific word he used to describe the cavalier attitude of the transplant community about a pandemic risk: denialism.

Church and Yang read everything they could about PERV, from its DNA structure to its potential infectivity. They then analyzed it themselves in a pig cell line (immortalized cells derived from pigs in the past). They determined that there were sixty-two copies of PERVs hidden in the DNA of these porcine cells. They then designed a CRISPR-guide RNA sequence to a critical portion of the PERV virus, to allow the Cas9 endonuclease to cut this portion out and prevent viral replication. They made sure this guide was specific to PERV and wouldn't disrupt any other genes in the pig cells.

These experiments were tedious and required many iterations, but were ultimately successful. After months of work, they were able to slice out a critical enzyme in PERV genes that prevented the intact virus from being transcribed. The success rate of the edits was not perfect—some cells evaded the CRISPR guide or underwent a recombination or repair of the edited gene after it was cut. But many of the cells showed near perfect disruption of PERV in every copy. The beauty of this process of gene editing is that not every cell needs to be perfect. After the edits, the cells are sorted and examined separately, and only those cells that reveal near 100-percent successful editing with minimal off-target events will ultimately be used for cloning animals.

In another set of experiments, they then tested whether the modified cells could eliminate transmission of PERVs to human cells. They placed either unmodified porcine cells or the porcine cells with PERV disrupted in culture with a human cell line. After a week of culture, they analyzed the presence of PERV DNA in the human cells. In the human cells mixed with unmodified pig cells, they identified one thousand PERVs per one thousand human cells. In the gene-edited pig cells, virtually no evidence of PERV infection was seen in the human cells after culture.

There were some limitations to these experiments. They were conducted using a pig cell line, and a pig could not be cloned from such cells. They would need to repeat their gene edits in primary pig cells in order to actually make pigs. Second, the human cell infection, prevented by the gene edits, was performed in cell culture, and not in an actual human. To this date, no human has actually been infected with PERV, and no one knows if PERV would cause any particular illness. So the importance of this edit remains theoretical.

Nevertheless, the paper describing this work, published in the premiere journal *Science* in November 2015, was received with great fanfare. They ended it by stating, "Although *in vivo* PERV transmission to humans has not been demonstrated, PERVs are still considered risky, and our strategy could completely eliminate this liability."[40] In addition, this paper was a huge advance in the use of CRISPR-Cas9 to perform gene edits. Prior to its publication, the maximum number of genes that had been edited at once was six. In these experiments, the Church lab edited sixty-two, without any obvious off-target effects. This illustrated the potential of editing any number of genes necessary to make pig organs acceptable in humans. Suddenly Tector's triple knockout pig, published earlier this same year, seemed rather banal.

* * * * *

In the first couple of years after the purchase of Revivicor, Martine and her team were sorting out Revivicor's personnel, collaborators, available pigs, and a small list of genes to target. But then, in 2013, CRISPR-Cas9 rocked the world. This didn't change Martine's vision, but it disrupted her list of goals. The previous five-year goals became one-year goals, and the more aspirational ten-year goals became achievable five-year goals.

Martine knew it was time to put together a team of prominent experts in gene editing. She describes her role as the person who can communicate the grand vision, but also the short-term goals and the day-to-day milestones. She can put the most effective teams together, whether they come from academia, industry, or regulatory bodies. She never settles on one strategy for success, knowing that the risk of failure would be too high. She believes in taking multiple shots on goal, with defined short-term milestones. If those milestones aren't reached, she will swiftly shut those efforts down and move the resources to other teams.

Once CRISPR became a reality, she reached out to Church, proposing a collaboration that would allow his team to perform gene edits in pig cells that Revivicor could in turn use to clone the animals. Martine also began a collaboration with David Sachs, supporting some efforts in his beloved mini-swine. She wasn't convinced that particular herd would be necessary, but she knew that Sachs was brilliant and that more shots on goal would be useful. There was another person she contacted, someone as famous as Church in the world of gene editing: Craig Venter. Venter, one of the fathers of the Human Genome Project, has been described as George Church with a better-trimmed beard. But there are some pretty major differences between the two. Whereas Church is beloved by everyone who meets him, Venter engenders a more controversial response.

* * * * *

Venter's personal story is legendary in the world of science. He grew up in California, not far from Silicon Valley. He was a terrible student, entirely unmotivated in school until he developed a fascination with science. By 1984, he was working at the NIH as a geneticist. It was clear to everyone around him that he was brilliant, but he was also brash, uncommonly driven, competitive, and not seen as a team player. He also gained the reputation of being motivated by money by attempting to patent genes that he and others were studying—an effort that failed to generate any patents but did generate some very negative feelings.

He left the NIH in 1992 and shortly thereafter had a major breakthrough. With a collaborator he had met at a scientific conference, he sequenced an entire bacterial genome just a few years after the Human Genome Project had been launched by the NIH and its international collaborators.[41] It occurred to Venter that he could sequence the human genome faster than the HGP. He saw this as an opportunity to patent many genes that he would be the first to identify, and also to stick it to the institution that frustrated him just a few years before. Venter partnered with a lab equipment company and raised venture capital money to start Celera Genomics in 1998, with the express goal of beating the HGP in sequencing the human genome. The two groups together announced the mapping of the genome in 2000, three years ahead of the target date.[42]

While Venter was credited for speeding up the process and inventing many new techniques for rapid gene editing, he also horrified scientists worldwide for his profit-driven work. Since then, Venter has continued to innovate—and continued to piss off those working with him. In 2005, he started a company called Synthetic Genomics, which collaborates with ExxonMobil to utilize modified microorganisms to produce clean fuels. He also succeeded, in 2010, in creating "synthetic life" by synthesizing a DNA molecule containing a bacterial genome, and introducing it into an empty cell.[43]

Venter has a lot of characteristics that would intrigue Martine. He is brilliant, brash, known for speed and efficiency, and prone to giving the middle finger to the establishment and any doubters. He was involved in big, outlandish projects that most people doubted were possible, but that had the potential to change the world. How could Martine not fall for someone who created a new form of life by engineering a bacterial genome? That project gets at the very definition of life, and the artificial boundaries we have placed on what it means to be alive.

In 2014, United Therapeutics issued a press release announcing that Lung Biotechnology Inc. and Synthetic Genomics ". . . have entered into a multiyear research and development agreement to develop humanized pig organs using synthetic genomic advances. The collaboration will focus upon developing organs for human patients in need of transplantation, with an initial focus on lung diseases."[44] Both Martine and Venter waxed enthusiastically about the importance of the collaboration, the project, and what the future would hold.

* * * * *

The idea of genetically modifying pigs to make them suitable for organ transplant in humans was the kind of project that Church could really sink his teeth into. Unraveling the genetics of what makes someone a human, or a pig, and studying what rewiring was necessary to cross the barrier between species was the kind of thing that Church loved. As a synthetic biologist, he had a different take on the potential than a transplant immunologist might. Simply modifying pig organs so they could function in humans was too limited of a goal. What really intrigued him was the possibility of generating *enhanced* organs. Church could picture organs that wouldn't be injured by the diseases that caused their failures. He could imagine organs that were resistant to human infections or other pathogens. He could envision organs that would never develop cancer, or would be protected from senescence and aging. He could even imagine generating organs that would be resistant to injury from extreme temperature, organs that could be cryopreserved and thawed whenever needed. These were the kind of challenges that excited the synthetic biologist in Church, and all of these goals seemed plausible, most of them already demonstrated in some form or another in living organisms. It became clear to Church, after reading about the collaboration between United Therapeutics and Synthetic Genomics, that if he wanted to design pigs for xenotransplantation, he would have to make it happen on his own.

Shortly after publication of the manuscript describing inactivation of PERV, Church formed a company named eGenesis, with Luhan Yang as the CEO. Church was sure to highlight the importance of their accomplishments with PERV and its relationship to the future of xeno, which he explicitly stated in an interview with the communications department of his institute at Harvard. "The presence of this type of virus found in pigs . . . brought over a billion of dollars of pharmaceutical industry investments into developing xenotransplant methods to a standstill by the early 2000s."

In the same interview, Church was even more definitive about the importance of their findings. "PERVs and the lack of ability to remove them from pig DNA was a real showstopper on what had been a promising stage set for xenotransplantation." He described their work as "an explosive leap forward in CRISPR's capability when compared to its previous record maximum of just six simultaneous edits." Yang got in the game too, in an interview with the Xinhua News Agency in October of 2015: "Our work dispelled the shadow PERVs cast on the field more than a decade ago when the virus was discovered, while renewing our faith in xenotransplantation."

The implications were that the field had stalled out and investigators were just waiting for someone to come in and figure out how to proceed. This was certainly not the case. Many of the xeno researchers were focusing on the immunological hurdles, but tremendous progress had also been made in the understanding and potential management of PERV if xeno were to proceed. Most importantly, it had been shown that PERV came in a few different flavors, and there were herds of pigs that harbored PERVs less likely to infect humans. This knowledge, in combination with ability to monitor for PERV DNA and potential antiviral therapy against PERV virus if it was to become a problem, had mitigated concerns about this virus in the minds of many in the xeno community. Church continued to think this was denialism.

Church and eGenesis weren't actually ready to focus on the immunologic hurdle. They had another challenge to address. Their 2015 *Science* paper was a proof of principle, all done in a cell line. They had to actually make a pig.

And make a pig they did. In September of 2017, the eGenesis group, with Yang as senior author and in collaboration with Church's Harvard lab, published an even more impactful paper in *Science*.[44] They first translated their findings in the pig cell line to primary pig cells, inactivating all the copies of PERV in the cells. This proved challenging and they had to work through various failed experiments, but they ultimately succeeded. They then used nuclear transfer to generate cloned pigs that had no active copies of PERVs. At the time of the publication they had fifteen healthy piglets, the oldest at four months.

To add to the import of the paper, and as a rebuke to the naysayers in the transplant community who were questioning the relevance of PERV, they performed a series of experiments examining the ability of pig cells to infect human cells. They demonstrated that pig cells in culture had the ability to infect human cells from a cell line in culture, and these human cells could then "pass PERVs robustly to fresh human cells that have no prior exposure to pig cells." There still was no evidence that living humans could become infected by PERVs, or that PERVs would cause any actual illness, but it was hard to read this paper and not be a little bit nervous about the potential.

Church conducted a confident interview with *Scientific American* that had to sound pleasing to the venture capital community.[45]

> "I generally hesitate to say we've solved a two-decade-old problem, but in this case, we have," he notes. So far the team has only made female pigs, raised in a lab. They are now repeating the process to engineer male pigs, which Church says he doesn't expect to be any more complicated. The next stage of the research, Church and Yang say, will be to essentially "humanize" the pigs—

modifying them enough that their organs can function in the human body. This involves immunological changes as well as making the tissues compatible and fixing blood-clotting issues. They have already begun such work and are writing it up for submission to a peer-reviewed journal, Church adds.

The publication had been preceded by a Series A fundraise of $38 million, primarily coming from large venture capital firms. Church never had trouble raising money.

7 TRANSLATING THE VISION

Xenotransplantation had been given new life. The discovery of CRISPR-Cas9 led to declarations that healthcare was entering an entirely new era, with "personalized" or "precision" medicine becoming buzzwords that rolled off the tongues of industry experts, investors, and healthcare leaders every time they took the podium. The timing couldn't have been better for Martine Rothblatt, Joe Tector, and George Church—the visionaries who were funneling endless resources into making xeno a reality. But in order for xeno to make it from the bench to the bedside, through the regulatory hoops and over financial and ethical hurdles, the predictions and innovations would actually need to be translated into reliable outcomes in animal models. For years, there was consensus in the transplant community that human trials could not begin until graft survival surpassed at least six months, maybe even a year, in life-sustaining transplants in primates. No one had come close to this. This final piece of the puzzle would require a new generation of xeno-pioneers, transplant surgeons or scientists who would harness the innovations of the visionaries to make the xeno-revolution a reality.

———————

"I got quite a backlash from my family. 'Why are you using this animal?' My father used to always ask me, 'Can you at least try using another animal?'"[1]

It may seem surprising that one of the premiere xenotransplant researchers in the world, Muhammad Mohiuddin, is a devout Muslim who grew up in Karachi, Pakistan, and wasn't even allowed to say the word "pig" without a rebuke from his parents. "'My mother used to make me gargle,' Mohiuddin told VICE World News. 'It was a big no-no in my family. It was forbidden in our home.' Mohiuddin would even accompany his father and brother to hunt wild pigs outside the bustling metropolis, in rural areas of the Sindh province."

When Mohiuddin was a youngster, he wanted to be a jet fighter pilot. But that dream was derailed when he was told his poor eyesight would prevent him from being able to do so. His interest shifted to engineering and biology, and he eventually made his way to medical school in Pakistan, becoming as fascinated with the heart as he once was with jet airplanes. He saw heart surgeons as the fighter pilots of the medical world. There was no opportunity for him to pursue cardiothoracic training in Pakistan, so in 1991, he made the decision to come to the United States. He secured a spot in the lab of Verdi DiSesa, a prominent cardiothoracic surgeon at the University of Pennsylvania who was conducting transplant immunology and xeno research. Mohiuddin was a talented and driven researcher, and it didn't take long for DiSesa to recognize this. He sat Mohiuddin down and shared some advice. Cardiac surgery was a great field, but DiSesa found himself so helpless watching his patients wither away and die waiting for hearts that would never come. Mohiuddin was so gifted in the lab—so persistent, with an uncommon ability to remain optimistic when others would get frustrated. If his goal really was to help countless people that were dying around the world, he shouldn't become a heart surgeon. He should instead focus his considerable talents on making xenotransplantation a reality.

He considered the immediate gratification he knew he would experience as a heart surgeon, versus the delayed satisfaction he would encounter in a research career. It was possible that he would not live to see the day when xeno became a reality. But Mohiuddin didn't accept that. In a short period, working exclusively with cells, mice, and rats, he had become a believer. He knew then that his life's work would be finding an unlimited source of organs for transplantation. He recognized the source would be pigs, although he wasn't yet working with the animal that was considered Haram. He recognized that at some point he would have to. (Mohiuddin would ultimately consult with religious scholars to get their opinion, and hopefully blessing, regarding the use of pigs. "The final consensus was that there's nothing greater in the eyes of God than saving the life of a human.")[2]

Mohiuddin immersed himself in the world of xenotransplantation. It would be his life's mission. After a couple of years researching transplant immunology in rodents, he conducted a fellowship in bone marrow transplantation and then human islet transplantation. He experienced minor success in small animal models of allotransplantation (in the same species) and xenotransplantation (transplanting organs from hamsters and rats to mice). Mohiuddin was becoming a familiar face in the small but growing xenotransplant community, presenting at international meetings and serving on panels. When he would present his long-term survival of heart grafts in rodents, he spoke optimistically about what this might mean for the fate of all those patients waiting in vain for organs. But he also knew that so much was possible in mice that wouldn't translate to humans. His dream was to run his own lab utilizing a pre-clinical model, with primates serving as recipients to pig organs. He didn't want to spend his entire career working with lab animals that could fit in his hand.

In 2005, an opportunity came knocking. Kevin Horvath, a heart surgeon at the NIH and director of the Cardiothoracic Surgery Research Program at the National Heart, Lung, and Blood Institute in Bethesda, Maryland, reached out to Mohiuddin. He was interested in ramping up a xeno research effort, and thought it was time to establish a preclinical primate model. He discussed the opportunities with Mohiuddin, which included large amounts of intramural funding from the NIH. Instead of applying for grants from the institution, the research would be reviewed every five years with recommendations on whether to continue the funding. Resources were extensive, and collaboration with outside industry would be encouraged. Mohiuddin jumped at the chance.

It took Mohiuddin a few years to put his team together, get his animal model up and running, figure out which pigs he wanted to use, and settle on a standardized immunosuppression regimen. His primary model would be the heterotopic heart transplant, placing pig hearts into the bellies of baboons. He initially obtained pigs from the federally funded National Swine Resource and Research Center, a University of Missouri facility funded by the NIH to generate transgenic pigs for biomedical research.

In that first five-year period, Mohiuddin and his team performed numerous transplants with a variety of immunosuppressive protocols and learned a couple of key lessons. First, it became clear to him that simply knocking out Alpha Gal was not going to be sufficient to overcome rejection of these organs in primates or humans. Second, standard immunosuppression that was working in human allotransplantation was not going to be enough for xenotransplantation. Even depleting T cells with antibodies at the time of transplant would not prevent rapid rejection of the xenografts. When T cells become activated by an antigen present in a transplanted graft, they receive a second activation signal that magnifies the immune response. In 1999, Allan Kirk demonstrated the ability of an antibody to this second signal (an antibody to the CD40-CD40 ligand pathway) in T cells to prevent rejection in kidney transplants in rhesus monkeys.[3] This was met with great excitement in the transplant field, but hasn't been translated to human transplantation. An early trial with the drug had to be stopped as it caused life-threatening clotting in human subjects. Newer versions of antibodies to this second signal are under development and now in human trials. Mohiuddin was able to obtain a few of these, and applied this strategy in his xeno model. David Cooper was also using second-signal blockade in his own transplant experiments in Pittsburgh.

After a few years Mohiuddin formed a collaboration with David Ayares and began using Revivicor pigs. The primary transgenic animal he focused on was an Alpha Gal knockout with a human complement regulatory protein knocked in. He performed xenotransplants using multiple iterations of standard and nonstandard immunosuppressive drug therapy, but always measured graft survival in weeks rather than months. He wasn't even matching the outcomes Cooper and Sachs had published with their Alpha Gal knockout. As his first five-year review approached in 2010, he supplemented his data with a bunch of cellular and mechanistic studies, hoping this would be enough to sustain his funding. Mohiuddin painted the most optimistic picture of the future he could. Then the reviews came in. They couldn't have been worse. The comments ran the gamut from "this line of research is not going to work," to "this is a waste of time and money." The formal recommendation was to shut the lab down.[4]

These were dark days for Mohiuddin. He had come to the NIH with such high hopes and expectations, was finally doing large animal heart transplants, and suddenly he was struggling to afford animals for transplants. He streamlined his lab, making sure every dollar spent was accounted for, and every employee was absolutely necessary. Then he did what every investigator in the country has to do from time to time—he begged. He was thrown a lifeline, albeit a small one, from Ayares at Revivicor. He was living on borrowed time.

Mohiuddin needed to try something different to improve his outcomes, and the clock was ticking. He had spent much of his career studying the response of B cells, a facet of the immune system that was primarily responsible for antibody production. He had originally hypothesized that the antibodies to the secondary signal on T cells would be enough to control the B cell response, but with the disappointing results, he decided to add another antibody that was specific for B cells (anti-CD20 antibody) at the time of transplant. By adding the B cell antibody, his graft survival improved from a median survival of ten days, up to a median survival of over a hundred days with one animal lasting 236 days, or eight months. This was the world record for a functioning xenotransplant when it was published in March of 2012.[5]

Mohiuddin wanted more. As he performed numerous iterations of his transplants, he noticed that the two things that were leading to graft loss were continued problems with antibody and clot forming in the graft due to platelet activation. Mohiuddin had numerous calls with Ayares, who added a gene edit to his pigs so they would express a human molecule that prevents clotting (human thrombomodulin molecule, or TBM). Now these pigs expressed no Alpha Gal, had a human complement regulator, and a human clotting regulator, all generated prior to the advent of CRISPR technology.

Mohiuddin performed heterotopic heart transplants in five animals. In February of 2014, he was able to report his first xenograft survival of a full year (still beating strongly at the time of the report).[6] Of the five animals, only one rejected the heart, at 146 days, while the others were still alive with functioning grafts. This was a major milestone in the xenotransplant community, and it came just in time. Mohiuddin was up for his next five-year review. When his evaluations came in, Mohiuddin had to laugh. The recommendations were to divert the majority of funds in the cardiac section of the NIH to the xeno lab. Mohiuddin was flying high.

He knew he could do better. With increased funds and personnel, Mohiuddin pushed forward at a frenetic pace, trialing different combinations and doses of immunosuppressive medications and transgenic pigs.

In 2016, he published his magnum opus in the prestigious journal *Nature Communications*, a report that catapulted him to the forefront of xeno research.[7] He demonstrated median heterotopic heart graft survival of 298 days, with one heart graft surviving 945 days. That's more than two and a half years! His drug regimen included a high dose of the anti-CD40 antibody that was given weekly throughout the experiment. As long as he kept the anti-CD40 antibody going, the graft functioned perfectly and no antibodies were formed in the blood of the baboons. But as soon as he stopped this weekly antibody, even after 900 days in one recipient, the baboons would reject the graft. Mohiuddin was disappointed by this, but hoped someday they could identify gene edits that would allow acceptance of organs even when immunosuppression was withdrawn.

His results had exceeded any of the targets ever mentioned as a prerequisite to human trials. A point of frustration was that the anti-CD40 antibody was not yet approved in humans. But he knew two things. First, newer, less pro-thrombotic version of this antibody were moving through human trials for autoimmune disease and would likely be approved in the near future. Second, there was a whole armamentarium of other strong immunosuppressive drugs that existed for humans that couldn't be used in primates, giving more options once the xenotransplants moved into the clinics. Mohiuddin was close to his dream of clinical xenotransplantation. He would now move onto the next step, transplanting the hearts into the chests of the recipient baboons, so they would be life supporting.

Mohiuddin was thriving at the NIH. He had gone from being considered a middling scientist following a pipe dream to the world leader in one of the most compelling fields in medicine. But he also faced limitations. There was no clinical cardiac transplant program at the NIH, so eventually he would need to find a different location to move the research into humans. Mohiuddin was getting more convinced every day that this was imminent, and he didn't want to miss his opportunity. The director of the cardiac research section was a heart surgeon, so between the two of them they were able to conduct orthotopic transplants of pig hearts into the chests of baboons, replacing the baboon hearts with the pigs. To do this they had to utilize cardiopulmonary bypass to keep the baboon alive during the transplant, which was no small task. They lost numerous baboons on the table as they were putting their team together and perfecting their techniques.

It was right around then that he got an unexpected call. "At this time, the President of United Therapeutics, Martine Rothblatt, along with the Chair of Surgery, Stephen Bartlett, contacted me and encouraged me to move to the University of Maryland to start a cardiac xenotransplantation program. I still remember Martine saying, "I hope you decide to move because you cannot discover new lands unless you are willing to lose sight of the shore."[8] She offered to support the program with a $24 million commitment.

This was the offer Mohiuddin couldn't refuse. Mohiuddin knew who Martine was. He was already collaborating with the company that she had bought a few years after he and Ayares had begun working together. But this would be something different, an opportunity that came at the perfect time. It didn't hurt that the University of Maryland Medical Center was less than forty miles down I-95 from Bethesda, and the institution had a twelve-year track record of xenotransplantation research funded by the NIH and United Therapeutics, conducted primarily by Robin Pierson.

On July 31, 2017 the University of Maryland put out a press release: "University of Maryland Medicine Establishes Nation's First Center for Cardiac Xenotransplantation with $24 Million Grant and Top Surgeon-Scientists." In the release it was revealed that Mohiuddin would be appointed as Professor of Surgery and Director of Xenoheart Transplantation. Mohiuddin was quoted as saying "We now have an opportunity to create the world's leading center for xenotransplantation research here at the University, leading to human trials within the next three years."

Martine's money came with milestones, yearly targets that had to be reached to keep the money flowing. This included constructing a clinical grade facility where pigs could be temporarily housed and taken to surgery for organ harvesting, meeting the strict guidelines that the FDA would demand for human trials. It also included specific milestones for baboon survival in an orthotopic cardiac transplantation from Revivicor pigs. Mohiuddin wasn't worried. With the support he would have at Maryland, including participation from the world-class cardiac surgery program run by prominent heart surgeon Bartley Griffith, he knew he could make it work.

* * * * *

Looking back in retrospect, it's hard to know exactly when the wheels came off at Indiana. Tector seemed to be flying high. He was running one of the largest transplant programs in the world. His patient and graft outcomes were excellent. People in need of transplants were flocking to Indiana for a chance to be saved by this larger-than-life character and his team. Up-and-coming transplant stars from around the world were vying for a chance to train with the master.

Tector was also becoming something of a celebrity scientist for his xeno work. He was a hot invite for grand rounds and plenary talks at international scientific meetings, and in virtually every talk, he would declare that human trials were imminent. He was in contact with the FDA, and he predicted that the first trial would begin in the next year or two. Tector was also savvy about the business opportunities that would accompany clinical xenotransplantation. In 2009, he had started a company to protect his intellectual property and commercialize his designer pigs. The original name was Xenobridge LLC, but eventually it would become Makana Therapeutics (Makana is the Hawaiian word for gift or reward). Tector was careful to file patents for the transgenic pigs he generated at Indiana, which were assigned to the Indiana University Research and Technology Corporation, with Tector as the inventor.

The lab was expanding in every facet. He employed scientists who had mastered cloning and gene editing, as well as a steady stream of residents from Indiana and across the country who wanted to spend a few years studying the science of xenotransplantation, many of them obtaining PhDs under Tector's tutelage. He brought his brother Matt on board, an expert in genetics, stem cells, and immunology. Matt comes across as a more mild-mannered, relaxed version of his brother with a quiet confidence, rather than the more boisterous approach his younger brother had adopted (although in family lore, apparently it's the opposite).

Around 2014, Tector began a collaboration that would be pivotal in his xenotransplant career. He was poised to make the transition from generating transgenic pigs to using them as donors in pig-to-primate transplants. The first step would be performing a crossmatch to look for antibody between any potential donor and recipient, just like he would do for a human transplant. Tector had the idea to test both primate blood (as primates would serve as his animal model) and human blood against the various transgenic pigs he had generated. Tector had access to plenty of human blood, but the primates were another story. He reached out to colleagues at the Emory Transplant Center in Atlanta, where a large National Primate Research Center was located. The Emory group agreed to provide samples from rhesus macaques and give input on study design.

Over the next year, the Indiana and Emory groups collaborated to test serum from humans, macaques, and baboons against the various transgenic pigs Tector had generated. The study suggested that each additional knock-out reduced the human antibody response to the pig blood.[9] It signaled to Tector that he needed to develop more sensitive crossmatching technology that he could use in the future to test potential recipients for their compatibility to his pig organs, techniques already available for analyzing responses to human antigens but not pigs.

But most importantly, it allowed Tector to form a relationship with a junior member of the transplant team at Emory, a surgeon named Andrew Adams. Adams had completed his PhD at Emory studying the immunology of transplant, and had recently finished his fellowship and started his own lab and clinical practice there. Although he was primarily involved in testing novel drugs in allotransplantation, he was ripe for a new set of projects. Tector was actively looking for someone with whom to collaborate for his planned pig-to-primate projects at the time. He had contemplated doing his primate experiments in house, but the cost and resources to conduct the transplants and care for the primates after transplant would be significant, particularly since there was not a national primate center in Indiana. Tector proposed to Adams that the two of them could work together developing protocols for xenotransplantation using pigs generated at Indiana and then transplanting them at Emory. Adams was game for it.

To the surgical residents training at Indiana at the time, Tector was a legend. They loved working for him and would do anything he asked to make his service run better. The junior residents who hadn't yet worked with him in the OR were told to find their way into his room to watch him do a liver. It was like "watching a symphony." The fellows, or advanced surgical trainees focusing on transplantation, were a bit more tortured, but remained loyal to their master. They knew they were getting the best training in transplantation available in the world.

Despite all of this, Tector's life at Indiana was becoming more complicated. He was a disruptor, always pushing the limits, growing and expanding wherever he could. There was no case he wouldn't take on, no transplant that seemed too complex, no organ that he couldn't find a home for. When the surgical ICU was overflowing with his patients, he just started putting them into the neuro ICU, the cardiac ICU, or wherever a bed might be open. When anyone questioned him about it, he would ask, "What do you want me to do? Let these patients die?" His Transplant Institute was taking over the hospital. He had so many dollars flowing through his Institute, paying for his clinical program and his research efforts, it was bound to get noticed. No other clinical leader at that institution had that much control of his revenues, and the grumbling was growing. Eventually leadership at the medical center changed, and Tector found himself reporting to less sympathetic ears.

Tector could always deal with the clinical side. He was used to fighting for resources and space. But when his lab support was threatened, that was a different story. Just as Tector's lab was finally generating cutting-edge pigs, he started to face accusations that too many resources were being funneled his way. Slowly but surely, Tector found that less of the money coming through his Institute was earmarked for research support, in violation of the agreement he had made when he became the director. In addition, some competitive university grants that his group had been awarded were withdrawn, at the discretion of the research leadership at the medical school. Tector knew he could stay on at Indiana as the director of the Institute and continue to run his massive transplant unit. But his dream of introducing the first clinical xenotransplatation program in humans was under threat.

By early 2016, just as Mohiuddin was submitting his seminal paper demonstrating survival of a xenoheart for more than 900 days, Tector was ready to find a new institution.

* * * * *

By the middle of 2015, as Tector's frustration at Indiana was growing, Martine decided it was time to take xenotransplantation to the next level. Novel transgenic pigs were on the ground at Revivicor. Mohiuddin was rapidly improving graft survival using Revivicor pigs as a collaborator at the NIH. His results were so impressive that the potential to move into human trials was no longer theoretical. But this was only part of the story. Martine and her small leadership team had been diligently meeting with Venter's team at Synthetic Genomics, generating a wish list of gene edits for an advanced pig the likes of which no one had ever seen before. Venter and his team of geniuses would soon provide Ayares with the edited cells that he would then use to clone the new animals. Martine's goal was to make one edited pig that could work for every transplantable organ, but she knew multiple iterations would need to be tested in primate models.

When Martine attracted Mohiuddin to an academic center with a strong clinical heart program, she envisioned a five-year plan with yearly milestones that would culminate in human trials. But Martine wasn't going to put all her eggs into one basket. Mohiuddin was a great asset, perfect to spearhead her efforts in cardiac xenotransplantation. But she still needed someone to drive experimentation in the kidney model. And of course she remained committed to making lung xenotransplant a reality, always thinking about what Jenesis might someday need.

Martine went back to her playbook that she used when she started United Therapeutics. She had the vision. She would then bring together a team of top-notch scientists in the field, those who had already distinguished themselves as brilliant and driven.

So who would be the other innovators for Martine to engage? In the discipline of lung transplantation, there really weren't many. Revivicor was already providing pigs to Pierson, a cardiothoracic surgeon who had spent his career committed to lung xenotransplantation. He had moved from Vanderbilt to the University of Maryland in the early 2000s and would be an obvious person to run the efforts in lung transplantation. Around this time, David Sachs was in the process of moving much of his lab to Columbia in New York City, where Megan Sykes was already running the xenotransplant efforts. Sachs, Sykes, and Kaz Yamada were brilliant researchers, and United Therapeutics would give significant funding to their labs to advance lung xenotransplant efforts. But that group would continue to focus on the use of the mini-swine that Sachs had been working with for more than thirty years, with the goal of achieving tolerance in the xeno model. As innovative as their work was, it wasn't likely they would fit into a regimented five-year plan with milestones set by Martine, and they wouldn't be interested in focusing on Martine's pigs.

There was one other person to consider. Joe Tector had become rather famous in the xeno world by this point. It was hard not to be impressed by his confidence, his seemingly endless knowledge base, and his consistent prediction that clinical xenotransplantation was right around the corner. Tector was making his mark in gene editing and pig cloning, an area where Martine had the world's most famous and capable gene editor, Craig Venter, on her payroll. The last thing she needed was another gene editor. But there was something interesting, different about Tector's strategy. Whereas Martine's group, as well as Church's eGenesis, were knocking in genes that would mute the immune response to pigs in addition to the Alpha Gal knockout, Tector was focusing almost entirely on knocking out carbohydrates to prevent any preformed antibody in the human recipients. Then he would rely on advanced crossmatching and immunosuppressive medications to suppress the immune response. This may have seemed inelegant in those heady days of CRISPR, but there was a certain simplicity to it. It would represent another shot on goal.

When Tector got the call from Alabama, he was somewhat surprised by the content of the conversation. He wasn't surprised that they called, as he was used to being recruited, but there were a few things about this offer that struck him as unique. First, the location. The transplant program at the University of Alabama at Birmingham was a powerhouse in the field, with high volumes and excellent outcomes. It was well staffed with little turnover in faculty or program leadership. They didn't seem to be in need of a new leader. More importantly, Tector wasn't aware that Alabama had any previous experience in the field of xenotransplantation. Why the sudden interest, and what did it have to do with him?

The University of Alabama houses one of the most advanced departments of cardiology in the country, with a pioneer in the management of pulmonary artery hypertension by the name of Robert Bourge. He was studying this rare disease as early as the 1980s and was one of the experts the Rothblatts sought out when Jenesis first received her life-threatening diagnosis. Bourge has played an important advisory role in United Therapeutics since its inception, serving on its Scientific Advisory Board. When Martine became focused on bringing xenotransplantation from the scientific arena to the clinic, Bourge made the case for making Alabama one of her flagship destinations. He floated the idea of creating a xenotransplantation program at Alabama with the goal of moving transplants into humans in a short and realistic timeframe.

Bourge and Devin Eckhoff, the chief of transplant at the time, put together a plan for the program, and they began negotiating milestones that would need to be achieved for continued funding. The organ of choice would be kidney, a much more realistic target than the uber-complex lung. The milestones were optimistic. Year one: get facilities ready for pig-to-primate transplants, finalize a conventional immunosuppressive protocol, make some decisions on the transgenic pigs to use. Year two, achieve satisfactory survival in the experimental transplants with conventional immunosuppression. Year three, do a bridge trial of pig kidneys in humans who have a lot of antibodies (put the kidney in for one or two months and then get them a human transplant), as part of a Phase 1–2 study. Year four, complete animal studies with the finalized transgenic pigs with conventional immunosuppression. Year five, start Phase 3 studies in humans. Each of these were measurable milestones with a distinct timeline. This would allow Martine to assess the progress, make adjustments, and cut off funding if milestones weren't achieved.

The very first milestone, the one on which the entire plan hinged, was recruitment of a director for the xenotransplant institute. Initial discussions about the institute were centering around an investment from United Therapeutics in the range of ten to twelve million dollars. When Tector's name was floated as a potential director, Martine upped the offer to twenty million, contingent on Tector signing on.

The recruitment of Tector to Alabama began in earnest at the end of 2015. Tector knew he would be giving up the clinical leadership of his transplant institute, his not-so-small fiefdom with a budget that rivaled many developing countries. He loved his clinical role at Indiana, but also knew that his long-term dream, his mission to bring xenotransplantation to the clinic, was being threatened by the new leadership at Indiana.

Tector saw the potential at Alabama, where a well-funded xenotransplant institute that he controlled could allow him to pour gas on his research endeavors. When he saw the initial proposal with the list of milestones, he believed that some were unrealistic. He did not see any way that pig-to-primate transplants could survive long term with conventional immunosuppression, regardless of how many gene edits were included. Every pig-to-primate experiment to date had shown that the costimulatory blockade pathway using drugs not yet approved in humans were necessary. He didn't see any great reason to perform bridge transplants. But what he did think was realistic was Phase 1 trials in humans in three years, and a full-scale Phase 3 trial in five.

Tector proposed some changes to the milestones. His revised targets fit the general timeline. The most significant modification in his proposal was the use of his knockouts for experiments rather than the more complex pigs that Revivicor and Synthetic Genomics were developing. Tector was not interested in working with any pigs but his own. As part of his recruitment, he had numerous conversations with Martine. Tector's impression of Martine was similar to that of so many others. She was a visionary, was committed to making xenotransplantation a reality. She made it clear to Tector that she wanted him to come to Alabama to head up this novel, state-of-the-art xenotransplantation institute and to be the one to bring xenotransplantation to the clinic. She was prepared to put serious money behind this effort. They shared the same dream, both believing it could be a reality and the time was now.

Martine didn't object to Tecor's plan to continue work on his own transgenic pigs initially, rather than the ones Revivicor was developing, as long as his outcomes could hit the milestone targets. He was convinced his pigs had the most potential, would be the easiest to produce, and would be the simplest pigs to advance through the regulatory obstacles that the FDA would deploy. Martine wanted xeno to be a reality to save her daughter and other people suffering from similar diseases. Tector offered the best chance to do that. It all made sense to him. He knew at some point they would have to come to a consensus on which pigs would be best for clinical trials. He was confident it would be his.

Once Tector received permission to start a multivisceral transplant program at the institution and to continue performing liver transplants, along with a grant from United Therapeutics for $19.5 million over five years, he agreed to come on board. His arrival at Alabama was announced at a press conference in April of 2016. It included speeches from the dean of the medical school, the chair of surgery, the chief of transplant, and of course Tector. Optimism was sky high.

Tector arrived at Alabama with some key members of his lab, including his experts in gene editing and pig cloning. He remained convinced that he had the right pig for human trials in his triple knockout, but he was also always thinking about the future. To him, the future meant knocking out more molecules that were targets of natural antibodies in humans. He had recently published that his triple knockouts reduced antibody load in 90 percent of the serum he had tested, but he still knew he could do better. He also wanted to design more sensitive and efficient cross-matching techniques, to better identify antibodies that could be a problem after transplant.

Tector had considered knocking in hDAF or another complement inhibitor, but he was hesitant to do so for one reason. He had engaged the FDA from the day he started generating pigs, and he was acutely aware that the regulatory bar would be much lower for pigs with genes knocked out than those with genes added. When a gene is knocked out, it's easy to show that the molecule in question is no longer present in cells. Then if healthy piglets are born, and the organ lasts for the required time in a primate after transplant, the FDA can be confident the transgenic pig is what they think it is. When a gene is added, it is much more difficult to confirm that the gene in question will be expressed at desired levels in the organs of interest, that it doesn't insert in a location that disrupts some other important gene, and that the added gene will be passed on to the next generation of pigs. Those animals may need to be cloned every time a new organ is needed, unlike the knockouts that tend to be stable after breeding. Tector was quite aware of the advantages a breeding program would provide for scalability. As good as Tector's team was at cloning, it remained a tricky, iterative, painstaking process. They would often have to implant upwards of seventy-five genetically modified somatic cells to yield one single live birth that harbored the knockout.

One of Tector's primary tasks at Alabama was to generate blueprints that met the specifications for an FDA-approved pig facility, hire a contractor, and build out a primate facility where the experimental transplants could be performed and the animals could be housed and cared for.

Tector wasn't the only major figure in the xenotransplant world that decided to make Alabama his sweet home. Just seven months after he arrived, David Cooper made his entrance along with members of his own lab. Cooper had been at Pittsburgh since 2004, and he also had served as chair of the Revivicor scientific advisory board from 2004–2011. Cooper enjoyed his time at Pittsburgh, but in a common refrain in the research world, the money was drying up. The chance to come to Alabama, with financial support from Martine and a vision to build an FDA-approved pig facility and move into human transplants, was too much to pass up.

At first glance, it might seem a bit redundant to have both Tector and Cooper as co-directors of the xenotransplant institute. In theory, it might have made sense, as Tector's lab had been focused on generating transgenic pigs and minimizing pre-formed antibodies, and Cooper's lab specialized in performing the transplants and taking care of the primates afterwards. But they both have big personalities, competitive spirits, and lifelong commitments to making xeno a reality. Conflicts were sure to arise. But with Tector directing much of his focus on his own knockout pigs, perhaps Cooper would be the ideal person to lead the efforts transplanting the Revivicor pigs, something he had been doing for the last decade in Pittsburgh. In addition, having two functional and competing teams may have been seen as a benefit. "Martine likes redundancy in everything she does," said one investigator involved in the Alabama transplants.[10]

* * * * *

It's hard to piece it all together, to put a finger on the moment things went south. On the clinical side, Tector suffered some growing pains. At Indiana, Tector had assembled the team, grown the department, brought in the money. He was used to showing up in the OR when the liver was coming off ice, sewing it in rapidly and precisely, and leaving the OR to go back to the lab. At Alabama, he was working with an entirely new staff that had their own way of doing things and that wasn't about to change, particularly for someone who wasn't their boss. As one surgeon there described it, "He came with so much force of will. He tried to break people down, break the institution down, thinking they would succumb to his way of doing things."[11] But it didn't work like that. Complaints started to filter in.

Tector thought the lab efforts were progressing well. He was advancing his crossmatching capabilities and learning more about his knockout pigs. He was characterizing a new knockout he had generated that, in addition to his triple knockout, also had a major protein involved in allorecognition removed (the pig version of the MHC class I). His work suggested that many humans have antibodies to this protein. His pig organs were being transplanted at Emory, and early results were looking promising.

But by Tector's second year at Alabama, life was becoming complicated. Only the first two years of funding from United Therapeutics was guaranteed. After that, his progress would be evaluated and compared to the milestones he had agreed to when he took the job, which included preparing for clinical trials or showing success with conventional immunosuppression. Based on the results of the transplants, there was pressure to focus on experiments with the Revivicor pigs, with the aim of moving them to clinical trials. He would not be able to ignore these demands, miss the milestones, and maintain his support at Alabama. Tector was hesitant to do this. His biggest fear was that his pigs would be shelved and left to die out at the farm while the more complex and sexy multiple gene-edited pigs became the focus of trials. He tried to negotiate for more control, more time, more money. But it was a dead end.

Tector's relationship with Cooper had become strained, and that was probably better than the dynamic that had developed on the surgical team. Tector's chairperson became quite familiar with the toxicity pervading the group. "Every time my phone rang at dinner or on the weekend my wife or friends would say 'uh oh, something must be going wrong in transplant.'"[12] Tector spent more time in meetings with administrators than in his lab or the operating room. By early 2019, Tector found himself with no operating room, a dwindling lab budget, and barely enough money to keep his pigs alive. A few months later, he was out of a job entirely. Sweet Home Alabama was no more.

* * * * *

Bruno Reichart was frustrated. He had just completed another orthotopic pig heart xenotransplant, sewing it into the chest of a baboon. The surgery itself had gone perfectly. That wasn't surprising, as Reichart had been involved in more than 1,100 heart transplants in his distinguished career. He had recently retired as chief of cardiac surgery at Ludwig-Maximilians University, the major university hospital in Munich, a post he held for over two decades. The German group Reichart worked with had fallen into the less-is-more camp when it came to transgenic animals. The pig Reichart was using was an Alpha Gal knockout with expression of the human complement inhibitor CD46 and thrombomodulin to prevent clotting. This was the same pig with which Mohiuddin had achieved so much success in his heterotopic heart model.

In its initial experiments, Reichart's group was supplied pigs by Revivicor, but more recently Reichart's pigs were generated at the Center for Innovative Medical Models, the pig facility in Munich where his research was conducted. His colleague Eckhard Wolf—a scientist with a background in veterinary medicine, animal breeding, and genetics—runs the facility and produces the pigs. It was Wolf who settled on these relatively simple animals, preferring to add single new modifications to address clinical problems rather than generate animals with multiple edits for theoretical benefit. "A smaller number of edits can be better controlled and measured, and their effects are easier to document."[13] This way if something goes awry with an organ, there is some chance to understand what the problem might be. "At some point, you are in a situation that you have no idea what an additional genetic modification does."

Using these pigs and the immunosuppression protocol developed by Mohiuddin, Reichart and his team had achieved similar success transplanting hearts into the bellies of baboons. As exciting as the results were, however, these hearts were not life-sustaining. Until someone could show that the pig heart could replace the baboon heart, no one could consider putting a heart into a human. Reichart figured that shouldn't be too hard for him, given how many transplants he had done in his career. But his initial attempts were met with disappointment. He performed a group of five pig heart transplants into baboons with standard preservation techniques employed when he removed the hearts from the pigs. He flushed out all the blood with preservation solution, cooled the hearts down on ice, kept them on ice while he was getting ready to sew them into the chest of the baboons, and then re-perfused the hearts once they were sewn in. Three of the animals were dead in one day, one died at three days, and the fifth lasted thirty days before it died. All of the animals died from severe heart failure, an outcome that has been seen in the majority of orthotopic heart xenotransplants, and is so common the entity even has its own name, perioperative cardiac xenograft dysfunction (PCXD).[14]

Reichart's group directed its efforts at solving this xenograft dysfunction. They were convinced that it had to be related to how the heart was preserved after it was removed from the pig. They decided to try a heart-perfusion system—once the hearts were removed from the pigs and flushed free of any blood, they were cooled and placed on an oxygenated pump that delivered preservation solution that included red blood cells, nutrition, and hormones. (This is different than the standard scenario, in which the heart is cooled and then sewn directly into the patient, or kept in a cooler until the recipient is ready for the implant.)

When these hearts were transplanted, three of the four in this group lasted 18, 27, and 40 days respectively. They looked and functioned better than those of the first group, but still suffered early failure. It was also notable that the hearts grew significantly in the baboons over that short period, a previously observed occurrence after xenotransplant. The hearts were harvested from juvenile pigs to be the right size for the recipients, but seemed to rapidly grow to the size they would be in a fully grown, six-hundred-pound pig. This would be deadly in the chest cavity where the heart is confined.

So Reichart's group made some more adjustments, adding on an immunosuppressive medication that prevents organ growth, managing blood pressure in the baboons to maintain the lower blood pressure pigs generally live at, and weaning steroids early after transplant. In a group of transplants following this protocol, two recipients lived for three months and still had normally functioning hearts when they were sacrificed (as specified by the study protocol). They repeated this protocol again, and two recipients were ultimately sacrificed with functioning hearts at six months. They did note that the hearts were functioning normally on the medicine preventing heart growth, but when they stopped this six months after the transplant, the hearts began to grow again. These findings were published in the premiere journal *Nature* in December of 2018, and were received with great excitement worldwide.[15]

This certainly was "a major milestone on the way to clinical cardiac xenotransplantation," which is how the German group described the work. They were surprised with how much the pig hearts did grow after transplant, and Wolf thought there might be a way to address this with a gene modification. By May of 2018, even before the *Nature* paper hit the press, Wolf had solved it.[16] He was aware of humans with a condition known as Laron syndrome, a hereditary disorder caused by genetic loss of function of the growth hormone receptor. A particular population of humans in Ecuador had two simple mutations in the growth hormone receptor gene. These patients were small in size but otherwise healthy. Wolf utilized CRISPR-Cas9 to generate pigs that had a similar growth hormone gene mutation as patients with Laron syndrome. The resulting pigs had a body weight that was 60 percent reduced compared to normal controls, and the organs were also smaller.[17] Reichart was optimistic that human trials were now within reach. He felt that in order to offer a pig heart to a human, he needed to do one more trial using these new hearts, and to keep a majority of the baboon recipients alive for a year. If he could accomplish that, he would feel justified offering these organs to humans. But not until then.

* * * * *

It would be Adams and Tector who would produce the next big windfall. They utilized one of Tector's knockout pigs, the double knockout (Alpha Gal and B4GalNT2). They could not use the triple knockout in the pig-to-primate model, even though that's the pig that the fewest number of humans have antibody against. As Tector showed previously, primates actually have more antibody against the triple knockout than the double, so they had to settle on the double knockout. No screened monkeys had completely negative crossmatches to these pigs to start, but they selected those with the weakest crossmatch. Using a similar immunosuppressive protocol that Mohiuddin had popularized, they reported a study in August of 2019 (just as Tector's time at Alabama was coming to an end, although the transplants were performed at Emory University) that had one animal in a group of six maintain kidney graft survival after transplant for 435 days, although the others were lost at earlier time points.[18]

This was the first report of a life-sustaining xenotransplant model with any animal surviving more than a year (Mohiuddin's protocol's long-term survival was not life-sustaining). Tector was thrilled that some animals lasted for so long, but knew he needed to do better. He came to a few conclusions. First, he hoped that outcomes in humans would be better, as he would be able to find potential recipients with entirely negative crossmatches prior to transplant. He would have various forms of immunosuppression to treat antibody-mediated rejection that don't exist for primates. But he also concluded that some form of human complement inhibition would be needed, to prevent any early antibody from damaging the graft. Tector was asked during a paper presentation why he wouldn't just add the human complement inhibitor to his pigs, something that had been done since the 1990s. Tector remained opposed for a few reasons. First, he was very deliberate and thoughtful about which genes he would delete. He had stuck with genes that provided no function and that had already been knocked out by evolution in humans. "Each of these genes that we have deleted is a gene that you and I have knocked out during the course of evolution. So, really, we are kind of talking about speeding up mammalian evolution."[19] He knew that would mean these modifications would not alter the physiology of the kidney and make it a poor organ for humans, since the humans had already disposed of these genes in their own evolution. Regarding adding genes in, he was trying to avoid that, as he was aware this was an issue that concerned the FDA. Tector also knew that certain viruses utilize human complement regulators as receptors that allow them to enter cells. This was even true of some viruses found in pigs. Although it was only a theoretical risk, Tector didn't want to add a transgene "which put viral receptors for important transplant viruses in the pig and make them a reservoir for new pathogens."[20] It would be like a Trojan horse, loading up a pig organ with virus and then putting it into an immunosuppressed human. Instead of gene editing, Tector identified a pharmaceutical agent that was an FDA-approved complement inhibitor, and began planning an experiment using his knockout pigs and treating the recipients with a short course of complement inhibition, a successful strategy that he would report in 2021.[21] Tector's mantra remained unchanged. Keep the gene edits simple. Iteration one would be knockouts only.

* * * * *

"CAMBRIDGE, Mass., Nov. 07, 2019 (GLOBE NEWSWIRE)—eGenesis, a biotechnology company utilizing breakthrough gene editing technologies for the development of safe and effective human-compatible organs to address the global organ shortage, today announced the successful completion of a $100 million Series B financing."

"With this new round of financing from industry leaders, eGenesis is well positioned to continue to advance the development of human-compatible organs to address the dire shortage in the US and around the world," said Paul Sekhri, president and chief executive officer of eGenesis. "The concept of cross-species organ replacement, known as xenotransplantation, has re-emerged due to recent advancements in gene editing led by eGenesis, and will become a safe and effective solution for the hundreds of thousands of patients currently on the organ transplant waitlist globally."

The lead investor was Fresenius Medical Care, one of the largest companies in the world providing dialysis machines and other care and pharmaceuticals related to kidney failure. Other investors included the Bayer's venture fund, the German pharmaceutical company, and some additional venture investment funds.

What was it about eGenesis and its progress since its formation in 2016 that got investors so excited? Well, at first there was George Church. They really didn't have any products at that point, but they had Church, the genius and darling of the venture capital world interested in the life sciences and investing in anything related to CRISPR. And they had the PERV-inactivated pigs that would serve as a platform on which all future edits would be conducted.

Whereas Tector's philosophy was to generate the simplest pig possible to achieve a negative crossmatch in humans, only utilizing knockouts of genes that humans had already shed via evolution, eGenesis would harness the most advanced gene editing in the world to modify the pigs in every way possible to increase their chance of being accepted. These two groups truly represent the two ends of the spectrum on the modern approach to gene editing, with Revivicor somewhere in the middle.

The eGenesis scientific team, led by Church himself, developed a technique to load all of their genes into a "cassette" that could then be inserted into the porcine genome using a site-specific insertion, allowing control of exactly where the genes go in the genome and how strongly they would be expressed. The technique also allows them to add new genes to the payload in the future, with all the genes delivered together into one location. They also planned to knock out the same three sugars that Tector targeted in his triple knockout.

eGenesis formed a partnership with Jim Markmann, the head of transplant surgery at the Massachusetts General Hospital and a rather prolific transplant innovator himself, and Tatsuo Kawai, a transplant surgeon and researcher who had previously worked in David Sachs's lab and continued to conduct tolerance and xenotransplant research in large animals. These two surgeons would conduct trials with the eGenesis pigs in the pig-to-primate transplants once they were available.

Towards the end of 2017, Luhan Yang made the difficult decision to leave eGenesis and return to China. The group was collaborating with a cloning facility in Hangzhou, China, and Yang decided to start her own company there, to be named Qihan Biotech. Church would remain a partner and advisor, and Qihan would focus on the same goal of generating pigs for transplantation. Unfortunately, in 2018 the pig population in China was almost entirely wiped out by the highly contagious African swine fever. Yang's current focus has reportedly switched cellular therapies. Reportedly.

eGenesis revamped its leadership team and hired a new CEO who took the reins in 2019. That same year they announced completion of the $100 million series B fund raise. That seems to be a lot of money for a company that had only published generating the PERV-knockout pigs. No preclinical transplant data had been reported. But they had Church and the most advanced gene editing strategy in the world. They had a collaboration with a prominent surgical team at the Massachusetts General Hospital. In the end, every biotech investor was looking for some big company that was going to change medicine by using CRISPR technology. You could do worse than betting on a unicorn started by the legendary George Church.

* * * * *

The nuns at the Catholic school in Buffalo, New York had seen this behavior before. A little boy who thought he knew better. "Most of my time there was spent being punished in the corner facing away from everyone, so I wasn't getting much out of it anyway."[22] Lucky for Bobby, and for the nuns, his relationship with the Catholic school would come to an abrupt end when his father, an engineer, would find a new job in Philadelphia. There would be no love lost between them. "They wrote in my report card that 'Bobby doesn't think the rules apply to him.'"

"Do you think people would say that about you now?" I asked him.

"I hope they would say that."

* * * * *

Bob Montgomery was the youngest of four boys in a close-knit family that he described as both happy and filled with mayhem. By the time Montgomery entered high school, his father became short of breath with the simplest of tasks. He initially figured he was simply out of shape and tried to push through it. But then he suffered his first "sudden death" as Montgomery calls it. He collapsed at home, but when he fell and hit the ground, his heart started again. He was diagnosed with a cardiomyopathy, most likely induced by a virus. He would spend more than half of the next two years of his life in the hospital.

Montgomery would spend many afternoons doing homework in his dad's hospital room. It was there that he saw the beauty of health care—the compassion, the desire to ease suffering, the teams working together to cure a patient's illness. But he also saw the limitations, the helplessness, and the inability to think outside the box. He was in the room when his mother asked the doctors, "None of this is working, so what's left to try?" As Montgomery recounts, "There was heart transplantation at the time, but this was 1976, and the doctors told her it wasn't available to anyone over fifty and it still didn't work that well anyway."[23] Montgomery's dad was fifty-two at the time. Montgomery remembers thinking, "Why doesn't it work? Why isn't this an option?" But he was fifteen. It didn't really matter what he thought.

After a year and a half of struggling with his illness, Montgomery's father had a massive heart attack. He was resuscitated but suffered significant brain injury and ended up in a vegetative state. Montgomery had to sit at his father's bedside for months until he finally died. Medicine truly had nothing to offer him over those last months of his life, other than a tortured and meaningless existence.

Montgomery was deeply touched by all of the compassionate and skilled people that put so much effort into caring for his father. He also wondered if there was more that medicine could have done for his dad—which primarily meant a heart transplant. Before his dad's illness, Montgomery saw himself becoming a veterinarian. But after the experience with his father, he started to set his sights on medicine. When Montgomery scrubbed in on his first operation as a medical student, he knew he had found his new home.

* * * * *

It was 2:30 a.m. when Montgomery's shrill pager broke the silence of the call room. He was an intern on the obstetrics and gynecology service at the Johns Hopkins Hospital in Baltimore, and figured someone had just gone into labor. But when he returned the page, he was connected to his sister-in-law. One of his brothers had just died. He was thirty-five years old, extremely healthy and fit, a successful lawyer living in Seattle. He was out waterskiing and had suddenly collapsed. The cause of death was a cardiac arrest. Montgomery was crushed. His initial feelings were for his deceased brother and the family he had left behind, a wife and his two young daughters. But as he recovered from the initial shock, Montgomery had another thought. This had to be genetic.

As the family mourned, Montgomery reached out to the medical examiner in Seattle. He needed his brother's heart. Montgomery made arrangements to have it sent it to a pathologist at Hopkins. He also still possessed the pathology slides from his dad's heart, which he brought down to the path lab. The pathologist looked everything over and told Montgomery it was definitely a cardiomyopathy rather than the more common coronary artery disease, and given the young age of his father's death and the even younger age of his brother's, it surely could be familial. Montgomery stood in the lab gathering his thoughts. He picked up his brother's heart from the laboratory bench and looked at it intensely. "I actually held his heart in my hands."[24] It wouldn't be the last Montgomery heart he would hold.

There were some benefits to being an intern at one of the finest hospitals in the world. He had access to some of the most advanced specialists and medical tests whenever he needed them. After some consultations, Montgomery found himself running on a treadmill in the cardiac catheterization lab with tons of wires running from his body to a bank of monitors. Within minutes, Montgomery's heart starting firing like mad, and the cardiologist ran in and hit the emergency stop button. Montgomery was having malignant arrhythmias, any one of which could have caused a cardiac arrest. It was clear at that moment that Montgomery shared the same hereditary cardiomyopathy that had just killed his brother, and his father before him. The one fortunate piece of news was that a surgeon at Hopkins had just developed the world's first implantable defibrillator. The defibrillator wouldn't prevent a life-threatening arrhythmia from occurring, but would deliver a shock if it happened, hopefully resetting the heart and allowing the normal contraction of the organ to resume.

In 1989, Montgomery became the first practicing surgeon in the world to have an implantable cardiac defibrillator. It had to be inserted directly into his heart, while his chest was open on the operating table. The power pack was as big as a twelve-ounce can of soda, and was buried under his skin through a separate incision in his abdomen. It was a debilitating surgery. But worse than the recovery was Montgomery's new reality. Could he return to his previous life, working long hours, taking care of sick patients, and conducting intricate and delicate operations where the very survival of his patients depended on his ability to get through the operation? In those first few months after the defibrillator was implanted, it "went off a bunch. It was so dramatic and debilitating." In this barbaric version of a pacemaker that now seems like a torture device, it would wind up, making a sickening sound, letting you know you were about to be shocked. When the defibrillator would actually fire, it was not subtle or gentle. "It was like getting struck in the chest by a two-by-four."[25]

After he recovered from the implantation, Montgomery met with his chairperson, the world-famous surgeon John Cameron. Montgomery was about to spend two years in the lab in Oxford, working with the prominent transplant surgeon and immunologist Peter Morris. Montgomery's meeting with Doctor Cameron was not to discuss a career in transplant, but whether he should consider leaving the field of surgery entirely. Cameron, a believer in Montgomery, suggested that he should go spend his time in the United Kingdom, learn the science of transplant, and they would see how he was doing when he returned in two years.

Montgomery and his pregnant wife were sitting in their flat enjoying their tea in the leafy, idyllic, and ancient apartment in Oxford when they heard screeching and then the inevitable sound of crunching metal and splintering wood, followed by a woman's screams penetrating the air. Montgomery was out the door before the cacophony had died down. The smell of burning rubber and oil filled his nostrils. It took a minute for his eyes to adjust to the scene in front of him. He saw a woman lying on the pavement screaming. His eyes scanned the street and he saw an upside-down car with its wheels still spinning and smoke all around it. He couldn't quite make out what the woman was yelling, but it sounded like something pertaining to a baby. He looked in the overturned car. The windows were all broken. The front seats were empty, and he leaned his head in the window and scanned the back seat. There he saw a baby strapped in a car seat crying.

Without thinking, he crawled in through the window and shimmied his way to the baby. He gently unstrapped the infant and lifted her carefully out of the car. As he lifted the child out, he wondered if the smoke permeating the air was a sign of a fire that was about to erupt and envelope the car. His heart was pounding as he felt the adrenaline pumping through his bloodstream. He crawled out, while somehow managing to keep the baby in the air and away from any of the broken glass and twisted metal that littered the area. As he exited the car, he could hear the police sirens approaching in the distance. He passed the crying baby to his pregnant wife. Just after he handed the baby off, he heard the wind-up sound, felt the hair on the back of his neck stand up, and realized what was about to happen. His defibrillator had fired in response to his racing heart. "Boom!" It fired again. He sprawled out on the pavement trying to catch his breath. He couldn't see anything, and felt a strong urge to vomit. "Boom!" It fired again. As his eyes rolled back in his head, he wondered if he had just died.

* * * * *

After this horrifying experience, Montgomery decided that he needed to take a more decisive approach to his own physiology. He recognized that the stress and adrenaline that he felt when he was climbing into that car was similar to how he felt when he was responding to a coding patient in the wards, or a trauma in the ER. His stress response had the potential to activate his defibrillator. "This isn't going to change. I'm going to have to change myself. I can't exist on adrenaline anymore. I can't put myself in situations where I could potentially get shocked. I changed my way of thinking about life."[26]

It would be nice to simply decide not to get stressed about things happening around you. Most people, however, are unable to just will that stress away. Montgomery had a secret weapon. He had a built-in biofeedback machine. The defibrillator. "It became a part of me and it was always part of me." Montgomery started his metamorphosis with a simple calculation. He thought to himself, what is the worst thing that could happen in any situation? The answer was that he could die. He saw that as a real possibility. But anything less than that was not worth worrying about. Particularly when he knew that worrying would increase the chance he would drop dead. This change in his physiology didn't happen overnight. It took time and effort, and each failure led to another horrific electric blow to the chest. But over time, he mastered his emotions. "I had to completely remodel my brain and not allow my body to react."

He returned to Hopkins after his time at Oxford, with plans to resume his training in and out of the OR. The first thing he and Doctor Cameron decided to do was ensure that no device in the OR would cause feedback in his defibrillator and shock him. He was hooked up to monitoring wires and brought to the OR, where the cardiologists could watch him as they activated all the different devices they might use during an operation. Nothing caused the defibrillator to fire. After that, Cameron gave him the green light. He was back in the program.

Montgomery spent the rest of his training mastering his emotions and his skills. After a major trauma or an operation with massive blood loss, fellow residents and fully trained surgeons would remark to him that he seemed so calm and unnerved, it was like he had valium circulating in his blood. But it wasn't valium. "Every time I went down to a trauma, scrubbed on an operation, got up to give a presentation, I would first talk my stress response away, mute the voice in my head. It always started with "what's the worst thing that could happen here? I could die. Anything less than that shouldn't be a problem at all. So let's just relax and take care of the problem.'"[27]

Montgomery excelled as a surgeon and a leader. He completed his training, which included a transplant fellowship, and came on staff at Johns Hopkins. Roughly ten years after returning from the United Kingdom, Montgomery would become the director of the transplant program at Johns Hopkins. His focus would always be exploring novel ways to get more organs to people who needed them.

* * * * *

Much of Montgomery's transplant career has been spent transplanting the untransplantable. His concentration has been on kidney transplant, where the waitlist includes more than one hundred thousand patients waiting for an organ. Half of those patients will never receive one, as they will become too sick waiting on dialysis for an organ that won't come in time.

In addition to growing the transplant division at Johns Hopkins and turning it into a world-renowned program, Montgomery is known for two groundbreaking advances that have changed the discipline. He developed and performed the first Domino Paired donation, something now called Kidney Paired Donation (or paired exchange).[28] It is simple in concept—say you want to give your sister a kidney but your blood types are not compatible, and I want to give my brother a kidney but our blood types are not compatible. How about I give my kidney to your sister and you give yours to my brother? He extended this to two-way, three-way, four-way, five-way, six-way, and eight-way domino paired donations. He also performed the first ten-way open-chain donation, where a humanitarian donor set off the domino paired donation.[29] In 2010, he was credited in The Guinness Book of World Records with performing the most kidney transplants in one day.

He was also the world leader in incompatible transplantation—or finding ways to override the immune system to allow transplantation across incompatible blood types or antibody barriers.[30] In other words, say I want to donate a kidney to my brother. When the crossmatch is performed, testing his serum against cells from my blood, it shows that he harbors antibodies that would attack my kidney. If we just do the transplant, the kidney would be rejected rapidly, just like what would happen if an unmodified pig kidney were put into a human. In the days before paired exchange, the center would turn me down as a donor, and my brother would be stuck waiting for a kidney from the waitlist. Montgomery and his team spent years devising a strategy of filtering the blood (a technique called plasmapheresis, similar to dialysis in which the proteins are filtered out of the serum) and giving strong immunosuppression to keep the antibody-producing cells at bay, and was successful in transplanting many of these patients with reasonable outcomes.

While the trajectory of Montgomery's career was undeniably upward, his personal life was filled with more ups and downs. As Montgomery was completing his training at Hopkins, one of his two remaining brothers had to undergo an urgent heart transplant. Montgomery had his brother's heart shipped to Hopkins to be compared to the other Montgomery hearts. Montgomery may well be the only person in the world that has held the hearts of three family members in his hand at once (well, two hearts and the pathology slides of his dad's heart). Montgomery's own heart had been behaving well now that he had achieved a Zen-like state, with few sudden electric shocks and no episodes requiring him to scrub out of an operation secondary to a cardiac event. Montgomery was resolute that no matter what happened to him, he wasn't going to let this disease define him in any way. He wasn't going to cut corners in his life or avoid any opportunities out of fear or caution. He didn't feel like he was just doing this for himself. He had three children now, two sons and a daughter, and his brother who died had two daughters. Montgomery knew his disease was hereditary, and feared it was passed down in an autosomal dominant fashion, meaning each child had a 50 percent chance of being born with it.

"I had to set an example for the rest of the family," he says. "I wanted them to know you could have this and still live a full life." His disease was liberating to him, as serious illness often is. It has allowed him to not sweat the small things in life, to think more about what really mattered to him and what he wanted to accomplish. "My mind is unencumbered with a lot of things I used to focus on. If you let go of that feeling of wanting to strive, things come to you more easily."[31] Over time, Montgomery became extremely comfortable with personal risk. It also affected how he dealt with his patients, talked to his patients about what they really wanted and feared. He was always thinking outside the box about ways to help more of them in the fashion they really wanted to be helped.

* * * * *

In 2017, Montgomery arrived in a remote part of Patagonia for his annual fishing and hunting trip with his sons. He was less than one year removed from his own professional transition from Johns Hopkins to his appointment as chief of transplantation at New York University, where he was recruited to rebuild a program that had fallen on hard times. Montgomery was still running full steam, both professionally and personally, and a hunting trip to Patagonia while reconstructing a transplant program in the city that never sleeps was on brand for him.

Shortly after arriving in Patagonia, Montgomery developed some flu-like symptoms. They seemed mild at first, and he chose to ignore them. Then, one night at the hotel, he developed shaking chills. He couldn't get warm as he huddled under the blanket, and after some hours of feeling like he was going to die, he arrested. One of his sons started doing CPR on him, and between that and his defibrillator, he came back to life. Montgomery doesn't remember much after this, but his shoeless son and the hotel staff carried him through the snow to their truck, performing CPR in the back until they got him to the tiny hospital that served Patagonia.

The staff took one look at Montgomery and said there was no way they could take care of him. An ambulance was called, and somehow he survived the five-hour drive to a slightly larger hospital. He had a breathing tube inserted into his airway and was placed on a ventilator. He was diagnosed with a severe pneumonia and spent three and a half weeks on the breathing machine in a medical-induced coma, lying on a stretcher the entire time. When he finally stabilized, he was airlifted back to New York. He couldn't talk or walk. He was being fed by a feeding tube. He was so weak that any time he tried to eat or drink, he would immediately aspirate into his lungs. Everyone taking care of him thought he would die, but he was absolutely set in his mind that he would recover. Less than three months later, he was back in the OR, performing kidney transplants.

A few months later, Montgomery and his wife, opera star Denyce Graves, were on Broadway, seeing the show *School of Rock*. They were about twenty minutes in when Montgomery experienced that familiar jumping feeling in his chest. Next thing he knew, he felt the two-by-four slam him in the chest. It didn't work. Montgomery passed out, and Denyce screamed. A nurse happened to be in the audience, and she laid Montgomery down and performed CPR. The code lasted a long time, long enough for the ambulance to arrive, the EMTs to take over. "The funniest thing . . . it's so New York, you're gonna love this! They immediately stopped the show, and when I woke up I was being put on a stretcher. They lifted it up, and I popped up and looked around. Everyone was standing. I waved and pointed. Everybody broke into an ovation, everyone clapping."[32]

Montgomery was back at work the next week. Despite all these near-death experiences, he was still too healthy to qualify for a heart transplant. After each arrest, his heart would recover enough to keep him going, and too much to move him up the transplant list. Unlike for his kidney patients, who could receive an organ from a living donor, that option didn't exist for hearts. It didn't help that he was blood-type O, and was a big guy (six foot one), making it even harder to find an organ. He would just plug along and hope for the best.

Then came Italy. Montgomery was invited to give a talk at an international conference on living donor transplantation in Matera, Italy, in the summer of 2018. Montgomery was sitting on the hotel bed, starting to undress, when he felt palpitations in his chest. At first it was just a few funny beats, but then it started to go faster and faster. He yelled out to Denyce, who was in the bathroom getting ready for bed. As she ran into the room, she saw Montgomery collapsing to the stone floor, landing directly on his face. He was unconscious, and blood was spraying out of a gash in his cheek. Finally, after sixty long seconds that felt like hours, his defibrillator fired, shocking him back to life. Denyce helped him stumble back into the bed. She called down to the desk for an ambulance, and held pressure on his face with a washcloth. His heart was going haywire at this point. Montgomery felt like he had a bag of worms in his chest. He endured a series of two-by-fours to his chest as his defibrillator tried to take back control of his cardiac rhythm. Every time it revived him, his heart went back into a disorganized, life-threatening cadence.

When they finally arrived at the tiny local hospital, Montgomery was met by a priest who gave him last rites. Montgomery suffered multiple arrests in the ER in Matera. As the physicians tried to attend to Montgomery, telling him he would be admitted for a long stay, it became clear to him that he was going to die there. He was just too complicated for that venue, or possibly any hospital at this point. He needed to get home.

The physicians in Matera thought Montgomery was crazy, that he would surely die if he tried to leave. The Italian physicians left the IVs in Montgomery's arms, helping him drape a long-sleeve shirt over them. They loaded him up with syringes of resuscitative medications that could help restart his heart if he arrested while in flight. Montgomery and his "team," his wife and transplant surgeon-friend who had been at the conference with them, boarded a flight from Rome to New York. Montgomery remembers waking up during the flight and seeing his friend staring at him. Montgomery couldn't help but think his friend looked oddly excited. Montgomery felt the need to say something. "The whole idea here is not to use these meds!"[33]

He made it back to New York and was quickly brought to the ICU at NYU. Most of the staff there had no idea that Montgomery suffered from heart disease. As they assessed his heart function, it became clear he needed a transplant badly. His heart was pumping at just a fraction of what it should have been. Montgomery was becoming short of breath just trying to get out of bed. They all wondered if he would get an offer before it was too late. Montgomery also struggled with the idea of taking a heart from someone else who might need it. He had made it to fifty-eight, way longer than he ever thought possible. Perhaps someone younger might benefit more.

Montgomery signed up for a new trial, offering hearts from donors who had died while infected with Hepatitis C, a virus that can affect the liver over time. Newly available medications that could eradicate the virus were now available, but their efficacy in clearing the infection after transplant was unclear. "I'll take any heart you can find," he told his team. "I don't care if the donor has a needle in their arm." On September 20, 2018, Montgomery received a visit from his cardiac surgeon. "We have a donor. Heroin over-dose, in their twenties, Hepatitis C positive." Montgomery didn't hesitate. "Let's go."[34]

* * * * *

When Montgomery was lying in that ICU bed at NYU before the transplant, wondering if he had waited too long to try to get a heart and feeling guilty that he might take a heart from someone else who was more worthy, he had a feeling of helplessness that he hadn't really experienced before in his life. He couldn't get the idea out of his head that he was waiting for someone to die, ideally someone young and healthy who died in some unexpected accident or drug overdose. "Waiting in the ICU, I kept thinking about this paradigm that we've been under in transplantation for so long, which is that somebody has to die for someone else to live," he said. "That came into focus in a new way when I experienced it myself. That was the moment when I said, 'We've got to figure something else out.'"[35]

It occurred to him that he really hadn't accomplished anything yet. His successes at paired kidney exchange and desensitization had been important innovations, and had helped a few patients, most of whom had access to living donor kidneys. But they were really just scratching the surface. They wouldn't do anything for the vast majority of patients sitting in the ICU hoping that someone's life would unexpectedly come to an end so his or her life could go on. They wouldn't help him. They wouldn't have saved his dad. If Montgomery survived, he was going to do something different, something much more impactful than squeezing out a few more transplants for a few more patients.

* * * * *

Montgomery's transplant went perfectly, and he was home in ten days. He felt better than he had in years, maybe as long as he could remember. He finally didn't have a sense that he was a sick person. His energy level was higher than he could remember. "It was such a long shot that I survived everything that I really began to think there was some purpose, that I still had a purpose. After the transplant, I was already thinking about what I would have to do to take that next step. It was like I was training for an Olympic event, and I had a new energy, a new focus."

A year before Montgomery's transplant, he had attended the Kennedy Center Honors gala with his wife. He had known that Martine Rothblatt would be there, and he sought her out before the event. Montgomery had been interested in xenotransplantation for years. He had attended the Arden House Xenograft meeting honoring Keith Reemtsma in 1989 when he was a resident in surgery. When he became a world leader in desensitization, he would often get invited to research symposiums and international meetings to share his expertise. The challenge of xeno using pig organs was primarily overcoming the natural antibody to Alpha Gal. Who better to consider novel strategies than someone who had championed overcoming antibody responses in human-to-human transplant?

Montgomery recognized early on that the sheer magnitude of the natural antibody response was massive, a thousand times what he could deal with in human-to-human transplant. But once Alpha Gal was knocked out in the early 2000s, he understood that xeno would become possible. He was interested in applying the techniques he had developed for desensitization in humans. So many of those techniques couldn't be used in the primate recipients, either because they were too unwieldy and technically difficult to perform in a primate, or because the drugs were not tolerated or effective in any species other than humans. "The work Rothblatt and her company had been doing dovetailed so nicely with the work I'd been doing and the work I wanted to do. I had so much of the transplantation knowledge, and they had genetically altered pigs."[36]

At the gala, Martine and Montgomery talked briefly, long enough to realize that they were two of the most interesting people in a room full of the world's most accomplished people. The next day they continued their conversation for four hours, focused entirely on xenotransplantation. Montgomery was convinced that xeno was closer to reality than so many of the scientists seemed to think. He didn't have to spend time convincing Martine of that. They were two unconditional optimists, neither of whom were afraid to try something new and risky, the more dramatic the better. They started putting some plans into place.

A few months after Montgomery's heart transplant, he was ready to go after his destiny. His purpose now would be to change the paradigm of recipients waiting for someone to die before they could get transplanted. It was xeno or bust. If it was up to him, he would have favored a trial in humans at this point. He himself would have been willing to take a pig heart when he was lying in that ICU, at least as a bridge, a temporary transplant until a human heart could become available. Montgomery understood the risk to this, and thought a trial in kidneys would be safer. Rather than keep patients on dialysis, he wanted to start a trial of kidney transplantation, where recipients would receive pig kidneys as a bridge to a human kidney. But the FDA was not ready to allow that. They wanted more data. They wanted longer survival in primates, using the exact pig that would be used in the human trial. They wanted more data on PERV and other infectious agents.

Montgomery and Martine brainstormed together. The xeno field was stuck in a rut. Researchers could do pig-to-primate studies until they were blue in the face, trying a new drug or antibody, or another gene edit, slowly improving survival in this animal model. But in the end, it was just a model. Some of the most important immunosuppressive strategies used in humans for decades were not even usable in the primates. They wanted to do something big, something that could pull the field over the hump, make it clear to regulators and the population at large that xeno was ready for prime time. But they couldn't just put a pig kidney into a human. Or could they?

As Montgomery was lying in that ICU bed waiting for someone to die, a thought came to him. He needed a brain-dead donor to give him a heart. What if that same type of donor could be used to benefit humanity in another way? Montgomery was aware that patients who were brain-dead were legally dead, based on the Uniform Determination of Death Act adopted as law in 1981. Given that legal status, it would be conceivable to transplant pig organs into brain dead patients. Montgomery was aware that there would be logistical challenges, but it seemed possible.

After Montgomery's transplant, he and Martine discussed how they might do this. They reached out to the organ procurement organization that serviced the New York area, and talked with donor families to gauge their reactions to this type of research. Montgomery's own institution had a committee already in place to address this type of research, termed the NYU Research on Decedents Oversight Committee. A protocol for the potential experiments was drafted, formally reviewed, and approved by the committee. The experiments would be expensive, but that wasn't a problem. United Therapeutics cut a $3.2 million check to NYU to support the project. The experiments would also be controversial, and were sure to be extensively covered by the aggressive New York press. Would the public be supportive, or would there be uproar when it was disclosed that a brash surgeon was sewing genetically modified pig organs into brain dead people?

The leadership at NYU put their faith in Montgomery. On July 10, 2020, it was announced that Bob Montgomery, just two years removed from a life-saving heart transplant, would become chair of the department of surgery. Montgomery would start his run at making xenotransplant a clinical reality in the city that never sleeps.

8 XENOTRANSPLANTATION IS THE FUTURE OF TRANSPLANTATION

After a thirty-year hiatus, the timing is finally ripe for xeno to exit the pre-clinical arena. Pig-to-primate animal models have repeatedly shown graft survivals far beyond any previously stated milestones required to consider human trials. Much has been learned about mitigating PERV and other infectious concerns, with strategies ranging from removal of PERVs, extensive monitoring post-transplant, and viral therapy available to treat any xeno-derived infection that is encountered. Strategies of gene editing have advanced beyond what anyone could have predicted a few decades ago, which will allow rapid iterations and improvements once data in human xenotransplantation become available. Xenotransplantation is the future of transplantation, but it's happening now. We are witnessing the reality of the dreams of so many in our field. This chapter will focus on xenotransplantation into humans, beginning in 2021.

———————

On Saturday, September 25, 2021, at 4:00 a.m., Montgomery opened a cooler and removed a kidney that had been shipped overnight from a Revivicor facility in Iowa. It looked so much like any of the more than a thousand kidneys he had transplanted over the last thirty years, with one difference: it was a thymokidney. The thymus from the pig had been implanted under the kidney capsule two months earlier by Revivicor surgeons, using the technique Sachs and Yamada had perfected years before.

On Friday evening, surgeons from Montgomery's team at NYU had flown to the Revivicor facility and performed the procurement, much like they would on a deceased human donor. The donor was a simple Alpha Gal knockout (now termed a GalSafe pig), the same type of transgenic animal that had first been generated by David Ayares using homologous recombination twenty years earlier. The kidney, flushed of its blood, was packed carefully on ice and placed in the cooler, the same cooler that Montgomery was now opening in the operating room in Manhattan just a few hours later. His "patient," a sixty-six-year-old female brain-dead recipient who was not a candidate to donate organs herself, was prepped and draped, with an anesthesiologist monitoring the airway and the ventilator. Montgomery had already made an incision at the top of the leg and exposed the femoral artery and vein. He sewed the pig artery and vein to the recipient artery and vein, released the clamps, and watched with wonder as the kidney filled with blood and turned a healthy pink color. The kidney had been on ice for seven hours and appeared to enjoy its first taste of human blood. Within minutes, urine squirted out of the pig ureter. "It was better than I think we even expected," he said. "It just looked like any transplant I've ever done from a living donor. A lot of kidneys from deceased people don't work right away, and take days or weeks to start. This worked immediately."[1]

Montgomery and his team left the kidney outside the body, perched on top of the thigh and protected by a sterile bag. A catheter in the ureter allowed close monitoring of the urine output. The output was voluminous throughout the entire study. Immunosuppression was just two drugs, standard agents that are used in all human transplantation. The recipient was followed for fifty-four hours, at which point the kidney was removed and then the patient was disconnected from the ventilator, allowing her heart to stop. All of the blood and urine tests performed during those fifty-four hours suggested perfect function of the kidney, and visual and pathologic analysis after its removal confirmed that the kidney was healthy with no sign of rejection.

The choice of kidney was interesting. Rather than using a genetically more complex transgenic pig, they settled on the simple Alpha Gal knockout. Montgomery shares Tector's philosophy that the simplest transgenic pig with just a small number of genes knocked out, genes that were deemed unnecessary and even disadvantageous by evolution in the human genome, would be safe and adequate for successful transplant. Montgomery also figured that the FDA would be comfortable with approving this type of pig for transplant. He didn't have to convince Martine of this. In December of 2020, the FDA had approved this exact pig for human use as a source of meat. It turns out that a small number of humans develop alpha-gal syndrome, a meat allergy that is acquired when ticks transmit alpha-gal molecules into a person's body after a tick bite, triggering an immune-mediated allergic reaction. Although Revivicor certainly wasn't in the meat business, they got their foot in the door with the FDA. No approval was yet forthcoming for organ transplants. But at least these transgenic pigs had an FDA-approved indication.

It was also interesting that Montgomery and Martine chose to use a thymokidney, the composite organ first conceived by David Sachs in the 1990s. Sachs's group has remained committed to the technique as a method to induce tolerance or at least mute the immune response towards the transplanted organ. United Therapeutics was also interested in this novel organ, and even trademarked their own version of it—UthymoKidneys™, generated from GalSafe pigs.

The initial results of Montgomery's successful pig-to-(brain-dead) human transplant were released to the prestigious scientific journal *USA Today*.

Within hours it was front page news in major newspapers across the world. The *New York Times* headline was typical. "In a First, Surgeons Attached a Pig Kidney to a Human, and it Worked."[2] Montgomery highlighted the magnitude of the experiment. "The field up to now has been stuck in the preclinical primate stage, because going from primate to living human is perceived as a big jump. There didn't seem to be any kind of incompatibility between the pig kidney and the human that would make it not work," Dr. Montgomery said. "There wasn't immediate rejection of the kidney." The long-term prospects are still unknown, he acknowledged. But "this allowed us to answer a really important question: Is there something that's going to happen when we move this from a primate to a human that is going to be disastrous?"

The reaction across the public was almost universally positive, and the excitement was palpable. The story dominated the news for days. Patients flooded transplant centers with phone calls asking about when they might be able to receive pig organs. PETA did release a statement condemning the experiment: "Pigs aren't spare parts and should never be used as such just because humans are too self-centered to donate their bodies to patients desperate for organ transplants."[3] But it was not accompanied by any real protests or movements.

*****

Montgomery didn't have any trouble convincing Martine to let him use the simple GalSafe pig in New York, but she was not one to keep all her eggs in one basket. Five days after Montgomery's pig-to-brain-dead-human transplant, the group at Alabama also performed a decedent xenotransplant. By this time, Tector had left the city of Birmingham for sunnier skies in Miami, and Jayme Locke, a prominent transplant surgeon and researcher, had taken the helm. Martine and her team had come up with their super-pig, a transgenic animal with the perfect combination of knockouts and knock-ins that would serve as their candidate organ for all xenotransplants. The group started with the same triple knockout that Tector had settled on (and patented). They then added two human complement regulatory proteins to prevent activation of complement after transplant (CD46 and hDAF). It had been noted for years that xenotransplants led to episodes of clotting in the blood vessels of recipients, so they added two human regulators of clotting (thrombomodulin and endothelial protein C receptor). They added two genes to reduce the human immune response (CD47, which blocks destruction by immune cells, and HO1, an anti-inflammatory gene). Finally, they deleted the pig growth hormone receptor gene, as Wolf and Reichart had done in Munich. It was not possible to test every combination of transgenic pig in a primate transplant experiment, as that would be prohibitively expensive and time consuming. They did, however, conduct an iterative process to narrow their choices down to something manageable, using an *ex vivo* perfusion system pumping human blood through transgenic pig lungs, with follow-up pig-to-baboon transplants. This massive endeavor was done in collaboration with Pierson at the University of Maryland. The final product was a pig with ten CRISPR-derived gene edits in total (hence called 10-GE pigs), and the cloned animals appeared to be healthy. It was noted that they didn't breed well, so every additional animal would have to be cloned, an expensive and cumbersome technique.

Locke and her team transplanted two 10-GE pigs into a decedent patient, again using a standard immunosuppression protocol currently used in humans.[4]

Upon release of the clamps, both kidneys perfused beautifully. The right kidney made urine after twenty-three minutes, but the left kidney was "more sluggish." The brain-dead patient was closed and maintained in the operating room for the next seventy-seven hours. He did experience multiorgan failure due to his brain-dead status, becoming more unstable as time went on. The right kidney made urine the first twenty-four hours, but petered out after that. The left kidney made minimal amounts of urine. The recipient's creatinine, a laboratory measurement of kidney function, failed to correct, indicating poor kidney function. Biopsies of the kidneys did reveal significant kidney injury.

The study did show that the kidneys, similar to Montgomery's experience, did not undergo hyperacute rejection by preformed antibodies. At the end of the study, no PERV infection was identified. It is hard to comment on whether the kidneys functioned or would have performed better in a healthy human recipient, given the short follow up and the instability of the brain-dead recipient. It is well known that after transplant, many kidneys do take a while, sometimes weeks, to "wake up" and become functional, particularly when transplanted into a sick recipient.

A couple of months after Montgomery's first decedent transplant, he performed a second one with similar good results. Montgomery published his results in *The New England Journal of Medicine*, arguably the most famous medical journal in the world.[5] At the end of the article, the NYU group broadcasted their next move: "An assessment of the durability of positive outcomes in this model, as well as adaptive immune responses, will require longer-term studies involving recently deceased humans or clinical trials involving humans."

Just a few months later, in June and July of 2022, Montgomery's group at NYU transplanted two separate xenohearts into the chests of two decedent recipients, monitoring the function of the transplants for three days each before concluding the experiments.[6] The hearts were from the 10GE pigs, and standard immunosuppression was used. The hearts functioned perfectly, sustaining circulation in these recipients without the need for any auxiliary mechanical support. This was the first example of circulation-sustaining pig hearts placed orthotopically into the chests of humans, proving genetically modified pig hearts were strong enough to support human recipients. For three days anyways. As an interesting footnote to this experiment, the lead surgeon who performed these transplants (Dr. Moazami) was the same person who sewed the (human) heart into Montgomery less than four years earlier.

At this point Montgomery and Martine were in intensive discussions with the FDA about a path forward in humans, and at the same time looking to perform brain-dead transplants with follow up of at least a month. They had moved out of the primate arena. But the FDA remained hesitant to greenlight a full trial in humans.

* * * * *

David Bennet Sr. was in serious trouble. He had spent the last two months in the hospital with a failing heart. By this point, he was bedridden. His heart was barely pumping strongly enough to keep him alive, much less to get up and walk around. He was started on medications to maintain his blood pressure, and when that was inadequate, a balloon had been threaded into the main artery coming out of his heart to augment its function enough to sustain his life. Even this proved inadequate. After multiple episodes of cardiac arrests and CPR, he was placed on extracorporeal membrane oxygenation, or ECMO. Essentially that means he was on a heart-lung machine that would take out his blood, oxygenate it, and pump it back in to perfuse his organs. He only had one chance for survival: a heart transplant.

But no heart was forthcoming. He was assessed by four programs, and about a week before he was placed on ECMO, he found out the decision. He was denied by all four. There was concern about how sick he was, how debilitated he had become. But the primary reason for his denial was his poor compliance. Prior to his admission to the hospital, he had missed multiple medical appointments and skipped prescribed medications, often not even filling his prescriptions. Given how limited a resource hearts are, and the importance of taking care of them to prevent rejection, the transplant centers, including the University of Maryland where he was currently a patient, informed him that he would not be placed on the transplant list. He was as good as dead.

After Bennett had been told about his denial, he had a visit from his heart surgeon, Dr. Bartley Griffith. "We can't give you a human heart; you don't qualify. But maybe we can use one from an animal, a pig," Griffith recounted. "It's never been done before, but we think we can do it." When Griffith recounted the story, he admitted that he wasn't sure Bennett understood what he was proposing, until Bennett spoke up. "Well, will I oink?" Griffith had numerous conversations with Bennett and his family over the next few weeks, making sure they understood the risks, the novelty—that while he thought it could work, it also could end in a spectacular failure. Bennett was game. He wanted to return to his life out of the hospital. He wanted more time to spend with his family, his five grandchildren, and his dog Lucky. He summed his feelings up in one short statement. "It was either die or do this transplant. I want to live. I know it's a shot in the dark, but it's my last choice."[7]

There was one potential roadblock to proceeding—the use of a genetically modified pig organ, along with a crucial anti-rejection medicine likely needed for a chance at a successful transplant, was not FDA approved. The Maryland Center for Cardiac Xenotransplantation had recently been in discussions with the FDA about a trial with these experimental organs, but were so far unsuccessful in getting approval. When they re-approached the FDA this time, the request was different. It was for the emergency approval of this single transplant along with the needed medication to save someone's life that had no other option, a process sometimes called compassionate use. On the evening of December 31, the approval came through, with a note that said "Good luck with the surgery!" 2023 would be the year in which the world's first xenotransplant from a genetically modified pig into a living human being would be performed.[8]

Griffith and Mohiuddin (his co-director of xenotransplantation at Maryland) still had a lot of work to do to make this happen. They needed to confirm that the hospital would pay for the transplant and the immunosuppressive medications. Given the experimental nature, it was certain that no insurance company would cover it. They needed to make sure everyone on the team that would take care of Bennett was on board and understood the nature of what they were doing. They needed multiple consultations with psychiatry, ethicists, and anyone else they could think of to document that Bennett understood the nature of what he was doing, and that he consented to moving forward. They needed to select the pig that would serve as a donor and finalize all of the logistics. How did the University of Maryland find themselves suddenly ready to perform something so earth shattering?

* * * * *

When Mohiuddin arrived at the University of Maryland in the summer of 2017, he was filled with optimism and flush with money, to the tune of $24 million. Mohiuddin understood the biggest limitation of his previous research, that the transplanted hearts were heterotopic, placed in the abdomen of the primate recipients and not life sustaining. This heterotopic model was much simpler, of course. In order to do an orthotopic transplant, he would need to place the primate on cardiopulmonary bypass, where the heart-lung machine would sustain the recipient while the transplant was taking place. This was a major endeavor, both surgically complex and quite expensive. Things would be much easier at Maryland, where they hosted a massive cardiac surgery service run by the world-famous heart surgeon and researcher, Bartley Griffith. With the well-developed infrastructure, world-class expertise in cardiac surgery, and extensive funding from Martine, Mohiuddin figured he would have the orthotopic model up and running by the end of the year.

That's not how things worked out. After a few initial failures, Griffith enlisted his entire human clinical transplant team to ensure that every aspect of the transplant was conducted by seasoned experts. The team had surgeons, perfusionists (who run the bypass pump), scrub techs, and nurses. The management of the bypass machine was identical to the protocol used in the human OR. The immunosuppression was the same as what Mohiuddin had optimized in his successful heterotopic heart transplants over the last decade. In the fall of 2019, they published their results. They had performed six consecutive pig heart transplants into baboons, and all six animals were weaned from the bypass machine. But in every case, hours after removal from bypass, the hearts began to fail, and ultimately the animals arrested. Survival was less than a day in all but one animal. That one animal was kept on ECMO and survived for forty hours. The cause of failure was perioperative cardiac xenograft dysfunction.[9]

Mohiuddin was devastated. Thirty years of work on xenotransplantation suddenly seemed like an exercise in futility. What good was it to publish all these papers and give all these talks around the world, when in the end all he could do was sustain the beat of a worthless muscle in the belly of a baboon?

Around this time, Reichart's group in Munich began presenting their own successes with orthotopic transplant of the pig hearts. Their group showed that once the hearts were removed from the pigs, they had to be maintained in a hypothermic (cold) heart-perfusion system that included oxygen and solution with hormones and erythrocytes (red blood cells). The preservation solution they utilized was patented by XVIVO, a Swedish medical technology company focused on *ex vivo* organ preservation using solutions and organ pumps. The company originally had a focus on lung transplant and had great success through a collaboration with the University of Toronto, but had now expanded to all transplantable organs.

This was just the kind of company that would intrigue Martine. Despite her best efforts, pre-clinical attempts at lung xenotransplantation had not seen the same success as hearts and kidneys. Although Martine was fully committed to making xeno a reality, she needed other strategies to advance the field of lung transplant. Working with Toronto, XVIVO had developed a system to perfuse human lungs outside the body to assess function and improve quality. At the same time, the company had optimized this heart perfusion system and patented solutions to improve cardiac preservation. A collaboration was formed with United Therapeutics, XVIVO, and the University of Toronto. Martine would now have access to XVIVO's lung perfusion systems to be used on discarded human lungs, and Mohiuddin would utilize their *ex vivo* cardiac perfusion system and solution for use with the pig hearts.

Mohiuddin worked feverishly over the next few years at mastering the XVIVO system and assessing its effect on heart function after transplant into baboons. There was a learning curve, and initial results were only marginally better. But as they got more facile with the protocols, results improved dramatically. The perfusion solution seemed as important as the oxygenated pump itself. It contained electrolytes and hormones, including adrenaline and cortisol. Unbeknownst to Mohiuddin when he first started using it, the solution also included small amounts of cocaine. This product would ultimately get FDA approval, but when they first started using it, Mohiuddin had to answer numerous questions about what he was up to.[10] Imagine the irony of a devout Muslim importing a cocaine-infused solution that he would administer to pig organs.

* * * * *

By the time Mr. Bennett was an inpatient at the University of Maryland, Mohiuddin and Griffith were putting together their data on a massive set of experiments comparing various transgenic pig hearts transplanted into the chest of baboons utilizing the XVIVO perfusion system. These were life-sustaining hearts, doing the same job they would be asked to do in a human. When they utilized the XVIVO-preserved hearts from the 10GE pigs, animals survived a mean of 223 days before they were ultimately sacrificed. One animal had a normally functioning heart nine months after transplant, breaking the record that Reichart's group had set a couple of years prior. To add to the excitement, there was reason to believe that in humans, where more sophisticated care and monitoring could be provided, these hearts might last longer. The other transplants in their study, using hearts with less gene modifications, had shorter survival.[11]

When the Maryland group reviewed these data, they all agreed that it was time to proceed with transplantation into humans. Xenoheart transplant survival was well beyond the milestone proposed to consider a human trial.[12] They approached the FDA to discuss moving into a small human trial. Griffith had a long list of patients who were waiting for heart transplants, half of them in vain. He knew many who would gladly sign up for a chance at life, even if it was from a pig.

The FDA said no. Not yet. They wanted more primate data. They wanted larger trials in which the vast majority of animals survived a year. They wanted all the donors in the study to be from the exact transgenic animal that would be used in humans, and all immunosuppression the same in every reported transplant. They wanted the animals to be housed in GLP, or Good Laboratory Practice, facilities, with very specific requirements for housing, cleanliness, access, temperature. Any results from experiments that were not conducted in a GLP facility would not be considered. These were stringent demands. The cost of each primate transplant was so high, and the length of time required to do all of them would stretch into years. In the meantime, the Maryland group asked, would the FDA allow them to start some small Phase 1 trials? The FDA said no.

There was another way. The FDA had a pathway termed "compassionate use," available when an experimental medical product is the only option for a patient with a life-threatening medical condition who cannot otherwise enter a clinical trial. When pharma companies have a medication or treatment in a trial, they are typically wary of allowing a patient to receive it under compassionate use. These patients tend to be extremely ill or otherwise high risk. They often have comorbidities that place them outside of the criteria for a trial. These characteristics, combined with the publicity that often surrounds patients trying to get access to a last-ditch unapproved treatment as they approach death, increases the risk for a bad outcome for a medicine that has very little room for failure if it is ever to be approved. But in the case of xenotransplantation, there were no active trials of solid organs that could be derailed by a single bad outcome. Despite Mohiuddin's impressive data in primates, there was a lot of risk involved moving to a human. A pig heart had never been implanted in a living human before. Would it be strong enough to support the circulatory demands of a full-grown recipient? There was no way to know until someone attempted it. After much discussion, they agreed it was worth a try.

* * * * *

David Bennett Sr. may not have fit the bill as the perfect patient for such a risky and high-profile transplant. The biggest strike against him was that he was extremely ill. He was bedbound for weeks. He had previously undergone a mitral valve repair, which would make any heart operation significantly more difficult. His heart was beating so poorly that he had a balloon pump inserted next to his heart, and when that didn't work, he was placed on ECMO. He was essentially on cardiopulmonary bypass in his ICU room.

An additional strike was that he had been turned down as a transplant candidate due to his history of noncompliance. A xenotransplant would require more follow up than any other transplant, assuming the recipient ever left the hospital in the first place. In addition to monitoring heart function and immunosuppression, any patient receiving an organ from a pig would need to be observed closely for any sign of PERV or some other xenovirus. If there were any early signs of such an infection, that patient would need to be isolated, and any other close contacts would need to be tested and potentially even treated. The idea that the first recipient for a xenoheart might be a non-compliant person was a major risk.

Nevertheless, these were the circumstances that left Bennett Sr. in a position to qualify for the transplant under the compassionate use pathway. He truly had no other option to survive.

* * * * *

Friday, January 7, 2022

The morning started earlier for Griffith than he had originally planned. His elective pig xenoheart transplant was posted on the OR board for 7:30 a.m. At 2:00 a.m., he was lying in bed, his head spinning with thoughts of what he was about to do. At seventy-two, he was one of the most experienced heart surgeons in the world. After more than a thousand heart transplants, he could do that operation in his sleep. He had been an innovator throughout his career, which began at the University of Pittsburgh, where he often collaborated with Tom Starzl himself. In those early years he had a front row seat as Starzl pushed the limits on what was possible in abdominal transplantation. He witnessed many "sneak attacks," as Starzl called them, when he would defy the administrators and regulators and any other obstructionists who tried to stand in his way. Now Griffith was going to take the next natural step that Starzl always believed would happen—using a pig organ engineered at the same company he had thrown a lifeline to two decades earlier.

Griffith dragged himself out of bed, careful not to disturb his sleeping wife, and went downstairs to his kitchen. He grabbed his large mug out of the cabinet, the one that is too tall to fit in the Krups machine. He pulled the stand out of the way and hit the button. "Next thing I realized, I had coffee all over the floor. I had forgotten to put the cup under," he told a *New Yorker* reporter.[13] "You get a bit wiggly, a bit superstitious." He asked himself, "Do you know what you're about to do?"

Around the same time, Griffith's co-director was getting about the same amount of sleep. A snowstorm had been predicted overnight, with snowfall estimates as much as six inches. Mohiuddin had an hour-long commute even when the weather was good, and he could only imagine what it would be during a storm. He opted to stay on the couch in his office. He spent much of the night watching the snow falling outside his office window, contemplating what he was about to take part in. He had spent the last thirty years of his life with one goal in mind. Now, in a few hours, he would finally summit his own personal Everest. Sleep would not be forthcoming.

By six in the morning, Mohiuddin was down in the animal facility adjacent to the hospital. He watched as the 10GE pig that had been shipped from Revivicor's facility in Blacksburg, Virginia was prepared for surgery. Mohiuddin was in charge of the team that would remove the heart and place it on the XVIVO cold perfusion system, where it would receive oxygen, red blood cells, nutrition, hormones, and of course that small amount of cocaine. He had done this so many times before. There was nothing different about this day. Yet everything was different. This heart would go into a human. Mohiuddin could hardly believe it. Would it work? Or would everything he had worked for his entire career end in total catastrophe? Well, he would soon find out.

He watched the veterinarian and his team bring the sedated pig into the operating room. It was a large animal at 110 kilograms. It was much larger than the pigs they used in previous experiments. A pig this size would have a heart large enough to support a full-grown man. Once the pig was secured on the operating table, and prepped and draped, Mohiuddin made the long incision in the skin over the pig's chest. He sawed open the sternum and placed his retractors. He stared down at the beating heart, pausing for a minute to reflect on the wonder he always felt when witnessing a beating heart. Mohiuddin began his dissection, gaining control of the blood vessels that supplied this heart with pig blood.

At the same time, Griffith was getting started in the nearby human operating room. He had visited with Bennett and his family prior to the surgery. Bennett asked him one last time if he was sure he couldn't get a human heart. With none forthcoming, Bennett was ready to move ahead.

Bennett was placed on the operating table, and the anesthesia team put him to sleep. His own heart was barely working by this point, and he was kept alive by the ECMO circuit that had been running continuously for six weeks. Griffith opened up his chest and placed his retractors. He stared down at the massive lump of a heart that was barely beating in Bennett's chest. It was so enlarged and dilated that Griffith knew it would be a mathematical challenge to sew in the much smaller pig heart. He would need all of his experience and ingenuity to pull this one off. He placed his cannulas in the aorta and cava, to allow him to go on bypass.

Mohiuddin arrived in the operating room with his perfused heart in tow. As they prepared the pig heart for transplant, Griffith placed his clamps and removed Bennett's human heart. He stared down at the massive orifice that he would connect to the pig heart. The mismatch in size was extremely large, but Griffith didn't panic. He cut out a wedge of tissue from the recipient orifice and sewed it back together so the orifice was smaller. He then proceeded to sew in the pig heart, cooling it periodically with XVIVO preservation solution as he worked. After tying his sutures, Griffith released the aortic clamp. The pig heart expanded and went from a pale color to pink, receiving its first taste of human blood. Griffith gave it a shock and it started beating beautifully.

Before the celebration could start, they noticed their first major problem. Bennett's aorta had dissected. The layers of the wall of the blood vessel exiting the heart had torn from where the aortic clamp had been placed, allowing blood to dissect into the wall of the vessel and compress the "true" lumen. The dissection had propagated all the way into Bennett's abdomen, down to where the blood vessels ran towards Bennett's legs. This was a major, life-threatening problem.

They rapidly cooled the patient down to twenty-three degrees Celsius (73.4 degrees Fahrenheit), to put all of Bennett's organs to sleep. Once he was cold, they injected more perfusion solution into the pig heart to stop it from beating. They stopped the bypass pump and arrested circulation entirely, which Bennett could tolerate now that he was cold. In this scenario, termed hypothermic circulatory arrest, cellular activity in the organs are minimized and circulation can be halted for as much as forty minutes, hopefully enough time to fix the problems and restart the heart. Griffith repaired the aortic arch dissection with an artificial graft, which fixed the portion of the dissection that was in Bennett's chest. He then had his vascular surgery colleagues come to the OR and deploy a stent graft into the abdominal aorta to hold the true lumen open.

Once this was completed, he rewarmed Bennett. The xenoheart kicked right back to life, without missing a beat. The heart function was excellent, just like a high-quality human heart would have performed. This aortic repair led to significant blood loss and the need for blood transfusions, but the heart went right back to work. They decided to place a temporary closure on Bennett's chest and kept him on the ECMO circuit to minimize the workload of the heart as they monitored its function. Eight hours after the operation started, Bennett was returned to the ICU as the first man in the world whose life was sustained by a pig heart.

Bennett's blood pressure remained stable in the ICU postoperatively, but his kidneys, which had been working prior to surgery, never regained function after the operation. He returned to the OR on Saturday (a day after the transplant) to have a stent placed in one of the arteries to his kidney that had been blocked by the aortic dissection, in hopes to revive one of his kidneys, but it didn't work. He would remain on dialysis indefinitely. Meanwhile his heart was performing beautifully, and he returned to the OR on Sunday to have his chest closed. His breathing tube was removed at the end of the operation, as he was strong enough to breath on his own. He would remain on ECMO until Tuesday mostly as a precaution. His cardiac ejection fraction was normal and his blood pressure was actually on the high side, requiring anti-hypertensive medications to reduce it.

On Monday, January 10, the University of Maryland published a press release. "University of Maryland School of Medicine Faculty Scientists and Clinicians Perform Historic First Successful Transplant of Porcine Heart into Adult Human with End-Stage Heart Disease." It included a picture of Dr. Griffith standing next to Mr. Bennett, who was sitting up in his bed staring into the camera. Bennett looked tired and had a tube in his nose, but he also looked very much alive. The story exploded. It was front-page news in every newspaper and news program in the world. As Griffith told the *New York Times* when asked how the pig heart was working, "It creates the pulse, it creates the pressure, it is his heart. It's working and it looks normal. We are thrilled, but we don't know what tomorrow will bring us. This has never been done before."

When Griffith was asked about the operation itself, he gave an answer that conveyed confidence and yet implied it wasn't entirely straightforward at the same time. "The anatomy was a little squirrelly, and we had a few moments of 'uh-oh' and had to do some clever plastic surgery to make everything fit," Dr. Griffith said. As the team removed the clamp restricting blood supply to the organ, "the heart fired right up" and "the animal heart began to squeeze."[14] The entire transplant community was electrified.

Daily updates on Bennett's condition and progress remained front-page news. The idea that someone was living and even thriving with a pig heart was mind-blowing to the public, who had no idea this was possible. Griffith and Mohiuddin were in demand for interviews by every news outlet in the world. When they weren't on the phone, in front of a television camera, or in the operating room, they could be found at Bennett's bedside or sitting by a computer reviewing his data. Bennett was hailed as a hero. He was able to speak to his son on the phone, to tell him how much he loved him. His number one wish was to get out of the hospital and see his dog Lucky. He felt he could get there.

Griffith remained optimistic about the performance of the pig organ. "That new heart is still a rock star," Bennett's doctor Griffith said Wednesday in a video recorded by the hospital. "It seems to be reasonably happy in its new host, beating strongly. I would say it has more than exceeded our expectations." All of the articles in the press were undeniably optimistic, painting a picture of a man who was on the brink of death and now was on a path to recovery. No particular details about his clinical condition were released to the press or any other publication.

The true story was a bit different.[15] Bennett's heart seemed to be the one organ that was working well. Every other organ system suffered problems. Twelve days after surgery, he developed severe abdominal pain, and a CT scan suggested some abnormalities with his bowel. He was taken back to the OR for an exploratory laparotomy (his belly was opened up). He had some angry-looking bowel, most likely a sequela of the dissection that blocked flow to that segment of his guts. They didn't have to remove any bowel, but he did have infected fluid that grew bacteria and fungus. He was placed on strong antibiotics, but since he was on so much immunosuppression, they knew this would be life threatening. He didn't tolerate feeding through his gut and had to receive nutrition through his veins. His weight began to drop, which was concerning as he was already malnourished at the time of the transplant. His medical management became increasingly difficult as the days went by. His blood counts and immune cells dropped so low that some of his immunosuppression had to be stopped.

Bennett was able to watch some of the Super Bowl in his hospital bed on February 12, 2022, with his physical therapist. A video was released of Bennett mouthing the words of "America the Beautiful" during the pregame show.

Forty-three days after the transplant, Bennett became unresponsive with a low blood pressure, and the breathing tube was replaced in his throat. He appeared to have a severe pneumonia. He was clearly suffering from infections, so his team opted to administer intravenous immunoglobulin, a risky treatment as it consists of pooled antibodies from healthy humans. Although this can support the immune system of sickly patients, it runs the risk of introducing antibodies that could potentially react with a pig heart.

He stabilized for a few days, but then on day forty-nine he became increasingly ill. He was returned to the operating room for another exploration of his abdomen, but this failed to reveal any fixable problem. At this point, his heart was thickened on ultrasound and beginning to function poorly. Biopsies of the heart showed some abnormalities. It was unclear if this was an atypical rejection or there was some other cause. In the meantime, some of his blood tests raised concerns about a porcine-derived virus—not PERV, but a pig version of the common virus CMV. This was surprising to the team, as the pigs had been monitored carefully for this particular virus and were not thought to be carriers.

He was placed back on ECMO and treated for the virus and also for rejection. Biopsies on day fifty-six were more suggestive of antibody mediated rejection. By day sixty, it became obvious that Bennett was not going to recover. His heart was failing, he was requiring massive support to maintain his blood pressure, he was maxed out on antirejection medications, and he was suffering from infections at the same time. His weight had dropped fifty pounds, from a starting weight of 187 pounds to a nadir of 136 pounds. He looked like an end-stage cancer patient. After discussion with his family, support was withdrawn. He died with his family at his bedside. He never did get to see Lucky.

Bennett's son, David, thanked the team of doctors for the "life-extending opportunity" given to his father. "Up until the end, my father wanted to continue fighting to preserve his life and spend more time with his beloved family, including his two sisters, his two children, and his five grandchildren, and his cherished dog Lucky," David Bennett Jr. said in a statement. Those "precious weeks" wouldn't have been possible without the efforts of Griffith's team, Bennett Jr. said. "We hope this story can be the beginning of hope and not the end," he continued. "We also hope that what was learned from his surgery will benefit future patients and hopefully one day, end the organ shortage that costs so many lives each year."[16] Bennett Jr. told the Associated Press in January that his father knew the surgery wasn't guaranteed to work, but he had no other options.[17]

Griffith released his own statement: "We are devastated by the loss of Mr. Bennett. He proved to be a brave and noble patient who fought all the way to the end."[18]

* * * * *

Bennett Sr.'s transplant was just the beginning. On September 20, 2023, six months after Bennett Sr. died, Griffith and Mohiuddin transplanted a second man by the name of Lawrence Faucette. Faucette, a fifty-eight-year-old Navy veteran and retired lab technician at the NIH, suffered from severe heart failure, but was turned down for human transplantation at multiple hospitals due to a long list of medical comorbidities. He was deemed too sick to undergo a human heart transplant. After consultation with many specialists at the hospital, Faucette agreed to go forward with the xenotransplant, hoping to buy more time with his family. His goals were simple—to push the field forward, and to get to enjoy a cup of coffee with his wife on the front porch of their family home.

As simple as that goal might seem, there were some cards stacked against him. Faucette's heart had stopped twice prior to the transplant, and he had to be shocked back to life both times, with a breathing tube in place when he entered the OR. Faucette received the same Revivicor 10GE pig heart that Bennett did, and thankfully his surgery and early recovery were much more straightforward than Bennett's. Within a few weeks of surgery, Faucette was seen working with physical therapy. At a month, although still in the hospital, there were no signs of rejection, and plans were put into place regarding the rehabilitation unit he would transfer to after some more recovery. But it wasn't to be.

Shortly thereafter, Faucette started showing signs of early rejection, and despite aggressive treatment, at six weeks his heart ultimately failed. Griffith and Mohiuddin were devastated. Faucette and his wife knew what he was getting into, never had false beliefs about the likelihood of a long-term success. But that doesn't mean they didn't hope for something different. Before Faucette died, according to a statement released by the University of Maryland, he spoke to Griffith and the entire transplant team. "Mr. Faucette's last wish was for us to make the most of what we have learned from our experience, so others may be guaranteed a chance for a new heart when a human organ is unavailable. He then told the team of doctors and nurses who gathered around him that he loved us. We will miss him tremendously."[19]

Griffith and Mohiuddin vowed to learn as much as possible from Bennett and Faucette, and to push on with their efforts. Despite putting on an optimistic face to the press and transplant community, the disappointment was obvious. So much would be learned from these two groundbreaking transplants, but both patients were dead after two months. Xenotransplantation was left with more questions than answers. One question loomed larger than any others. Were we really ready to make the jump to humans?

* * * * *

When the news was released that the first genetically modified xenoheart was conducted on Bennett Sr., Bob Montgomery was asked how he felt, both as a xeno-researcher, and a heart transplant recipient with an inherited family illness that would lead to many more Montgomerys needing hearts. "It was stunning. It was incredibly inspiring and exciting, and my nieces and kids called me. It was very personal in that way."[20] Montgomery was a believer in the potential for xeno and had thought it was long past time to conduct human trials. His expectation was that the outcomes would be better in humans than in primates, given the higher level of care that could be provided, the plethora of medicines that have been developed to manage rejection and in particular antibody-mediated rejection, and the ability to find recipients without any pre-formed antibody prior to transplant, a challenge in the primate population. Yet, the first two patients had died so quickly.

The experience with xenotransplants into the decedent humans had been a remarkable success, but those recipients were only followed for a couple of days. He needed some way to test the outcome of a xenotransplant in a human model that he could follow for an extended period of time, long enough to convince the FDA, the public, and ultimately himself that a life-sustaining pig transplant could be successful enough in a human to move to a clinical trial.

Could he possibly use the decedent model for a longer trial? There were so many unknowns with this idea. First, it was unclear that a brain-dead patient could be sustained on a ventilator for weeks or more. Even if that was successful, could a xenotransplant keep working in a recipient that was suffering all of the organ dysfunction that typically accompanies brain death?

Would they learn anything from such a model? Finally, Montgomery struggled with the ethics of keeping a brain-dead patient on a ventilator for a prolonged period of time.

In the end, the family of a fifty-eight-year-old brain-dead man who was ineligible to donate his organs stepped forward, hoping to make his untimely death meaningful. On July 14, 2023, Montgomery and his team transplanted the simple GalSafe thymokidney into this brain-dead patient. Standard FDA-approved immunosuppression was used, and the patient was followed for two full months before the kidney was explanted. The kidney functioned beautifully for the duration of the experiment. There was one early rejection episode that was treatable with standard approved medications, a critical finding that had not been accomplished before in a xenotransplant from a pig to a human.

The patient's family was with the team every step of the way, grateful for the opportunity to advance the field of transplant and save lives in the future. At the end of the two-month trial, the kidney was removed and sent for analysis. It looked perfect. "It's a combination of excitement and relief," Dr. Robert Montgomery, the transplant surgeon who led the experiment, told the *Associated Press*.[21] "Two months is a lot to have a pig kidney in this good a condition. That gives you a lot of confidence for next attempts." A working pig kidney in a human at two months using standard immunosuppression was as much as anyone could hope for. The fact that this was achieved with an organ that had a single gene modification, knockout of Alpha Gal, was even more surprising. It was unclear what role the pig thymus tissue may have played in this outcome. Montgomery and his team were more confident than ever that the time for human trials had come.

* * * * *

On Saturday, March 16, 2024, the xeno-kidney (and eGenesis) finally had its day. The team at Massachusetts General Hospital led by Tatsuo Kawai transplanted an eGenesis kidney into a sixty-two-year-old man who was living on dialysis after a failed human transplant a few years earlier. Richard Slayman had previously undergone a kidney transplant in 2018, after having spent seven full years on dialysis, performed by Kawai and his team at MGH. His kidney lasted five years but ultimately failed. He returned to dialysis in 2023, and since then he had not been tolerating it well. His ability to dialyze was deteriorating and his doctor feared he would not survive long, certainly not long enough to receive another kidney transplant that would take years to find. When he was approached with the opportunity to receive a pig kidney through the compassionate use pathway, he considered the risks, and put his trust into his care team. "I saw it not only as a way to help me, but a way to provide hope for the thousands of people who need a transplant to survive."[22]

The kidney he was offered was the most genetically edited organ that had ever been generated—a pig kidney with sixty-nine gene edits, including fifty-nine PERV elements inactivated, three carbohydrates disrupted, and seven human genes knocked in to block complement activation, clotting in the kidney, and inflammation in the kidney after the transplant. It was also from a Yucatan Mini , similar to the swine that Sachs had chosen for his own experiments. Although this kidney had never been used in a human, Kawai and his colleagues at eGenesis had recently published a major paper in *Nature* analyzing its use in a large series of non-human primates.[23] They reported better outcomes with these advanced pigs than with the simpler triple knockout (of the three carbohydrates); one primate that received this organ had a life-sustaining kidney still functioning at 758 days. That's more than two years! (It's important to note that while the survival outcomes with the eGenesis pigs were impressive in this study, it still remains unclear which gene edits are needed to achieve prolonged survival. Other groups have published similar outcomes with the other transgenic pigs currently being investigated. Nevertheless, the results with the eGenesis pig were clearly excellent.)

The surgery on Slayman went smoothly, and the kidney began making urine right away. He was maintained on a similar immunosuppression protocol used in the second Maryland heart case, including the costimulatory blockade medication not yet approved by the FDA. The first week of Slayman's recovery was as easy as his first transplant in 2018, but after a week he began experiencing pain over the transplant and a worsening of kidney function. A biopsy was performed, and much to the surprise of his team, it showed a simple early T-cell mediated rejection, the garden-variety rejection we commonly see in human-to-human transplant (xenotransplants tend to have more problems with antibody in preclinical models). Slayman responded to a standard rejection treatment consisting of steroids and an antibody to T cells, and his transplant quickly recovered.

Slayman was discharged home two weeks after his transplant, with excellent kidney function. He was thrilled. "This moment—leaving the hospital today with one of the cleanest bills of health I've had in a long time—is one I wished would come for many years," he said in a statement issued by the hospital on April 3, 2024. "Now it's a reality." At Slayman's five-week visit, his kidney function was essentially normal. A planned follow-up biopsy showed no ongoing rejection. No antibodies against the pig organ were identified. He was noted to be weak and had suffered some weight loss. But he was well enough to stay out of the hospital.

* * * * *

Just days after Slayman went home, Montgomery's team got back to work. They identified a patient who clearly met the criteria for the compassionate use pathway. Lisa Pisano was a fifty-four-year-old woman who presented to NYU with a failing heart and kidney. She was so sick that she suffered a cardiac arrest in the hospital and had to be revived by CPR. She stabilized, but was deemed too sick to undergo a combined heart and kidney transplant. Her heart was so weak that she would need a mechanical device, termed a ventricular assist device (VAD), inserted into her chest to help her heart function. Because she was on dialysis, however, she didn't qualify for the VAD. That invasive treatment would only be approved for a patient who was a candidate for a combined heart-kidney transplant. She was stuck between a rock and a hard place.

After Pisano was turned down for the combined transplant, Montgomery talked the case over with Nader Moazami, the cardiac surgeon who had transplanted the pig hearts into the decedent patients. They brainstormed about how to save Lisa. They couldn't place a VAD in her if she was destined to be on long-term dialysis, but she couldn't get a human kidney transplant without a better heart.

What if Moazami placed a VAD in Lisa, and after she stabilized, Montgomery could follow with a pig kidney xenotransplant? They both agreed that it was Lisa's one shot for survival, would qualify for the compassionate use designation, and would be ethically justifiable for Lisa as her best and only option. They talked it over with Lisa and her family, and after much consideration she agreed to it. She wanted to live, but if it didn't work out, she would take comfort in the idea that her effort might help someone else down the road.

After emergency approval from the FDA, Moazami placed the VAD on April 4. She recovered for a week, and on April 12, Montgomery performed the pig kidney transplant. He used the same GalSafe thymokidney he had placed in the decedent a year before. The kidney made urine right on the OR table, eliciting cheers from the operating room staff. Montgomery was elated. This operation was the first VAD kidney transplant of any kind ever performed, representing yet another first for the team. Given the novelty of it, improvisation was required in those first few days after transplant. When Lisa's urine output dropped off shortly after surgery, they simply turned a dial on the VAD control system to increase the circulation of blood from the heart to the kidney, and the urine started flowing again.

One week after the transplant, Pisano took a walk with the help of a walker. Her kidney function was entirely normal. Montgomery found the experience of watching Lisa walk around the hospital with her augmented heart and pig kidney to be transformative. His entire career built up to that moment. Not just his career, but his entire life. He could draw a line from the months he spent doing homework at his dad's bedside in the hospital, watching him die a slow death from heart failure, to present, sitting at Lisa's bedside. He saw his own journey with heart failure, the many cardiac arrests and shocks and reprogramming his physiology to become comfortable with risk and stress, as a journey that is finally coming to its destination.

He spent the early portion of his career squeezing out as many organs as possible from people who had died, or maximizing living donation. But now, finally, he could see the different path. He could visualize the new paradigm, where patients dying of organ failure in ICU beds would not have to wait for others to die untimely deaths. The new paradigm would be something so beautiful. Hope would be engineered and bred, available whenever needed. In his mind, there would be a day in the near future when no one would die of organ failure waiting for a transplant. Transplants would be offered to the millions of people who wouldn't even be considered for this life-saving therapy today. As Shumway said so many years ago, xenotransplantation is the future of transplantation. And that future is now. At least in Montgomery's mind.

But the elation wasn't to last. Just under eight weeks after his transplant, Mr. Slayman suddenly died. Although the cause of his death was initially unclear, it was ultimately announced that he died of an unexpected cardiac event, with no signs of rejection, infection, or other dysfunction in his xenokidney transplant. His xenokidney was found to be entirely normal on explant pathology. His death was distressing to the entire xenotransplant community, as it was hoped that even if his kidney failed, it could be removed and he would be returned to dialysis. But that wasn't the case. His death was too sudden.

Forty-seven days after Lisa Pisano's transplant, her kidney stopped functioning and was removed. Lisa lived a few more weeks with her VAD in place and undergoing dialysis to replace her kidney function, dying on July 7, 2024—almost three months after her xenotransplant.

* * * * *

As the dust settled on the flurry of pig xenotransplants into humans, the xeno community took stock of what had just occurred. The Maryland transplants proved that a genetically modified pig heart could support the human circulatory system. Though it remained unclear what exactly led to Bennet Sr.'s and Faucette's deaths, everyone agreed that if they hadn't been so sick to start with, the outcomes might have been better.

The two kidney transplants done at Massachusetts General Hospital and NYU caused even more excitement initially, perhaps because Slayman was discharged home and Pisano, who underwent a combination of procedures never before attempted, was filmed taking a walk in the hospital. So many questions were left unanswered, but at least one thing was certain: the public was ready for attempts at clinical xenotransplantation.

There were no massive protests or death threats comparable to the aftermath of the Baby Fae transplant. Transplant labs weren't ransacked, animals weren't set free, private records weren't pilfered and released to the press. The animal rights groups were rather muted. Peter Singer himself, the man who wrote the bible on animal rights in the 1970s, was even quoted as saying he supported efforts at xenotransplantation. This surprised me, and I did reach out to him for clarification. "First, 'support' is too strong, maybe 'not oppose' would be better . . . I would not oppose the use of pigs who, as you say, are treated with respect, as individuals, and provided with what they need to live good lives. The reason I would not oppose this is that I would direct my advocacy against raising pigs in factory farms . . . and slaughtering them for ham or bacon, which don't save anyone's life, and in fact, according to WHO recommendations, are life-shortening.'"[24] That still seems a major departure from the atmosphere in the 1980s and 1990s.

These initial transplants had seemingly little effect on the FDA in regards to a timeline for human trials. Caution remained the word of the day, which is hard to argue with given the ultimate outcomes of the transplants. Investigators continued to meet with the FDA leadership searching for approval of small trials, and the response was consistent. The FDA continued to request more animal data, better outcomes, and consistency in immunosuppressive protocols.

* * * * *

The xeno world went quiet for the next five months. Leaders in the field continued to project cautious optimism, still predicting trials in the near future. If healthier patients could be considered in an FDA-approved clinical trial, perhaps the outcomes would be much better. Although Tector remained optimistic, he was more convinced than ever that xeno should only be trialed in patients with negative crossmatches, which might require knocking out more targets.

His lab continued to generate novel pigs with this goal. He published an opinion paper in *Transplantation* touting how far the field has come, but stating "there is still too much early graft loss from antibody-mediated rejection to surge ahead with clinical efforts."[25] In the article, he proposed that we would need newer pigs with fewer xenoantigens, extensive testing of these pigs in non-human primate models, and improved pre-transplant testing for antibody prior to moving forward with clinical trials. This must have frustrated him to write. This modern-day pioneer, who for years had been calling for trials in humans, voicing a call for restraint—that had to carry a lot of weight. The leaders of the xeno community embraced his message and all agreed to go back to the laboratory.

Or not. On December 17, 2024, news of another kidney xenotransplant splashed across the front page of every major newspaper in the country. It was performed, unsurprisingly, by Bob Montgomery at NYU in New York. The recipient was a fifty-three-year-old woman from Alabama named Towana Looney. He was assisted by Jayme Locke, his previous trainee at Hopkins who had recently relocated from the University of Alabama to New York to join her old mentor. Looney was a previous kidney donor herself, having donated a kidney to her mother in 1999. Unfortunately, her remaining kidney failed from high blood pressure, and although she went to the top of the wait list due to her previous donation, she had antibodies in her blood that made it almost impossible to find a compatible kidney. She spent eight years on dialysis, with no offers forthcoming. When Dr. Locke initially mentioned the idea of a pig kidney, Looney jumped at the idea. Dr. Locke had numerous conversations explaining the experimental nature, the risks, and eventually the outcomes in the recent recipients. None of that deterred Looney, who just asked, "where do I sign?"[26]

On November 25, 2024, Looney received a Revivicor 10GE pig kidney, rather than the simpler GalSafe pigs previously used. The immunosuppression protocol was based on conventional strategies, using all FDA-approved medications, similar to what they used in the decedent experiments. The kidney worked right away—urine squirted out shortly after the clamps were removed and the kidney was perfused with blood. She left the hospital in eleven days, and at three weeks had a minor rejection episode that was easily treated. On January 25, it was announced that she had become the longest living recipient of a pig organ transplant, surpassing two months. Her kidney function was entirely normal, she had been out of the hospital for more than fifty days, and was looking forward to traveling back home to Alabama in the near future.

"I'm a superwoman," she told the press. "It's a new take on life." After her transplant, Looney spoke to many waitlisted patients who were wondering if they, too, should consider a pig kidney. Although she was careful not to tell them what to do, she encouraged them that there are more options than just waiting for someone to die. "I want to give courage to those on dialysis," she added. "It's not easy, and it's not the only option. There's hope." Montgomery shared her excitement. "If you passed Towana on the street you wouldn't have any idea that she's the only person in the world who's walking around with a functioning pig kidney. That's a big deal." "It does seem futuristic," he went on. "It does seem like something I wouldn't see and be such a big part of my lifetime."[27]

Looney was able to return to her home in Alabama but, a little more than four months after her transplant, her creatinine began to rise. She returned to New York, where she was diagnosed with rejection. After considering everything Looney had been through, and the severity of the rejection, the kidney was removed on April 4, 2025, four months and nine days after it had been transplanted. Looney recovered well from the surgery, and returned home, back on dialysis but thankful for the opportunity, the hope that she had received. In Looney's own words, "For the first time since 2016, I enjoyed time with friends and family without planning around dialysis treatments. Though the outcome is not what anyone wanted, I know a lot was learned from my 130 days with a pig kidney—and that this can help and inspire many others in their journey to overcome kidney disease"[28]

* * * * *

On February 3, while Looney's kidney was still functioning, the hope had become official. United Therapeutics announced FDA clearance of its Investigational New Drug Application for the UKidney Xenotransplantation Clinical Trial. In the announcement, the company specified that "the trial will start in mid-2025, beginning with a cohort of six transplants at two centers. There will be a 12-week waiting period between the first and second transplants. After the initial cohort reaches at least 12 weeks post-transplant, safety and efficacy data will be reviewed." If results are positive, the trial size will increase to fifty patients in a multicenter study. The donor will be the

10GE pig, the same one Towana Looney received. This trial is considered a combination Phase 1/2/3 trial (or a "phaseless" study), and success with this trial could lead to FDA approval of the 10GE pigs for clinical transplantation.

That same day, eGenesis revealed that it was approved for a three-patient kidney transplant trial under the compassionate use pathway. The first of the three was performed on January 25, and the recipient, Tim Andrews, was a sixty-six-year-old who had been on dialysis for two years. It was estimated based on his blood type and other clinic factors that he had a 9 percent chance of receiving a human kidney in the next five years, and a 50 percent chance of being removed from the list or dying related to his health status and comorbidities. Andrews's immunosuppression regimen included co-stimulatory blockade, the still-experimental medication currently in human trials that has been required in the majority of pig-to-primate studies. Andrews will be followed for six months, and, as long as he does well, two additional patients will be transplanted with eGenesis pigs. Although this is not a true clinical trial, it certainly represents progress for eGenesis and the world's most edited pig. At the time of this writing, Andrews has just passed his eight-month milestone post-transplant, and in light of that result, eGenesis just received word that they will also be approved for twenty additional patients in a multicenter trial after the first three have been completed. His kidney function remains excellent, and he has been enjoying a robust life outside the hospital. On June 16, 2025, Andrews was joined by his transplant team at Fenway Park in Boston as he fulfilled a lifelong dream, throwing out the first pitch at a Boston Red Sox game. When he was asked if he was more nervous before the transplant or before taking the mound at Fenway, he gave the expected answer. "I'm more nervous to throw out the pitch."[29] (The pitch wasn't half bad.)

Will Tim Andrews break the sixty-five-year record for a xenotransplant set by Keith Reemtsma and Edith Parker in 1963? We won't know until the fall of 2025. But now there is hope. That's all anyone really wanted, anyway. And it's finally happening—clinical trials will begin in 2025.

* * * * *

So, this is the point of the book where I will make some predictions for the future. First, I will comment on what the next few years might look like (which seems a fool's errand, given that by the time you read this, I may have already been proven wrong). By the time this book is out, United Therapeutics/Revivicor and eGenesis will be well into their trials, perhaps done with the first six kidney transplants.

Although United Therapeutics has not announced which two centers would conduct the transplants, it is certain that NYU will be one of them, with Montgomery at the helm. If there is success with these first six pigs, then the trial will expand to fifty more at multiple centers. I am betting on enough success to proceed to the multicenter trial, by which I mean at least some of the patients will have sustained kidney transplant survival of more than a year.

I also predict eGenesis will complete their twenty-patient trial with the PERV-inactivated pigs. Tatsuo Kawai will likely perform the transplants in the eGenesis trial at Massachusetts General Hospital.

There are some differences in the strategy of gene edits between the pigs from United Therapeutics/Revivicor and eGenesis, but I predict that both pigs can be successful. For the first set of trials, patients will likely require long-term co-stimulatory blockade of T-cell function to prevent rejection, which means experimental drugs will be used in the trial. United Therapeutics/Revivicor has attempted to conduct their transplants using conventional immunosuppression, but I predict that this regimen will be inadequate to prevent early rejection and graft loss, and co-stimulatory blockade agents will have to be added to their protocol. A number of these co-stimulatory blockade agents are currently in Phase 3 trials at the time of this writing, so it is possible some will receive FDA approval prior to the multicenter trials.

I still hold out hope for a trial with one of Tector's pigs. But it's hard not to feel like he has fallen behind a bit. Perhaps Tector's smaller company just can't compete with the behemoths that United Therapeutics and eGenesis have become. But based on Tector's most recent publication and personal correspondence, he harbors concerns that the currently available pigs require too much immunosuppression and still suffer injury from antibody deposition. He has a new pig up his sleeve that he predicts will perform better than the current generation of transgenic donors. Even if Tector's pigs get a later start, I still believe they will have their day in the clinics. Remember, there will be multiple iterations of pigs before it is all said and done.

It will be critical that the recipients are robust and healthy other than their kidney failure, so they can tolerate the significant rejection crises that will almost certainly occur. It will be equally imperative that these patients are selected to be the lowest possible immunologic risk, with minimal preformed antibody and nearly-negative crossmatches. In terms of outcomes, I do believe that some (but not all) of these recipients will achieve more than a year of graft survival, but will require continued high-dose immunosuppression and will need to be monitored closely for infectious complications.

Although initial trials will occur in the United States, it is also possible that a different country could move into the clinic in the next few years. I have written about some of the efforts in Germany, and other countries such as Japan and South Korea also have active research programs in xeno, although their pigs are generally modeled after the pigs being produced here.

One country that could surprise us is China. It is hard to know what milestones have been reached in that country, although there have been publications describing the generation of transgenic pigs and a few decedent transplants, including one with a liver and one with a lung. In a recent report, surgeons from a hospital in China's eastern Anhui Province announced the successful transplant of a portion of a transgenic pig liver into a living patient performed on May 17, 2024.[30] The recipient was a seventy-one-year-old man who was undergoing a liver resection for a large liver tumor. The surgeons removed the tumor with a large portion of his liver, and then implanted an auxiliary pig liver to bridge him until his own remnant liver regenerated enough to sustain his life. Specific details about the procedure, the immunosuppression, and how long the liver was expected to last were not included in the report. It was described that the pig had ten genes edited, although it is unclear which genes were manipulated. In March 2025, it was reported that a female patient underwent a gene-edited pig kidney transplant at the Xijing Hospital of the Fourth Military Medical University in Xi'an, and is currently doing well. I search my news feed virtually every day for an announcement about a larger Chinese xeno trial that has been conducted, but no information is available about the specific gene edits or immunosuppression being used.

As for the heart, I believe that, over the next few years, more heart transplants will be conducted under the compassionate use mechanism, or perhaps as a bridge to a human heart in a patient that isn't a candidate for a VAD or mechanical heart. I predict that true clinical trials in hearts will follow success with kidneys.

It is unlikely that any xeno trials involving pig liver transplants will be considered anytime soon, as the preclinical data has been quite poor. But there has been a resurgence of interest in liver perfusion for patients with acute liver failure that might have a chance to recover function in their native livers. eGenesis has recently received FDA approval to enroll a select group of patients in a trial using their genetically modified pigs, and other trials are sure to follow.

In the near term, I believe that gene-edited pigs will receive FDA approval as a short-term bridge for patients that can't tolerate dialysis while awaiting human transplants. It might be more interesting, however, to think further into the future. Down the road, more complex pigs will be generated that will dramatically improve outcomes of xenotransplantation, reducing the need for extensive immunosuppression and improving the longevity of these organs. That is when the world of healthcare will be thrown on its head. Some of the gene edits will be knockouts of targets that our immune system might naturally recognize. Others will be immunomodulatory, to suppress the response of these immune cells when they do recognize the pig organs. I predict that the second generation of transgenic pigs will allow conventional immunosuppression to be sufficient after xenotransplantation, and it is at that point that pig organs will rival human organs. This will take some time, multiple iterations, and a few cycles of preclinical trials using primates as recipients followed by human trials. This generation may also employ potent tolerance strategies envisioned by Sachs and his team, potentially allowing dramatically reduced immunosuppression and improved survival outcomes.

These organs will function as well as human organs, but will still require at least some immunosuppression, and recipients will suffer many of the side effects our patients today experience. At this point, we will be able to transplant everyone on our waitlist, but the scope of transplant won't be significantly different. We will still limit the types of patients that can truly tolerate and benefit from transplants. It is the next generation of pigs that will transform our world. This is when we will be able to create bespoke pigs, matched to the genetics of specific recipients. When a patient is found to have a failing organ, we will send some of their blood to a lab, where a genetic analysis will be conducted. Edits will be performed in a pig cell, and then that cell will be used to clone a novel pig for that recipient. Six months after that pig is born, the organs will be ready for transplant. Less than a year after the diagnosis, a bespoke organ will be ready for transplant. Minimal immunosuppression will be required. Transplant will become something different, something more akin to the field of longevity. Replacement parts will be available for those that need them, when they need them. Millions of patients will benefit from these organs.

This will not be the end of it. The generations of pigs that follow will include genetic modifications that allow organs to last longer, organs that are resistant to cancer, those that can tolerate extremes of temperature and pressure, be resistant to infection, require minimal nutrition, and blood flow. These will be perfect for when we relocate to Mars. I know, this sounds like science fiction. But as recently as the 1950s, so did basic organ transplantation. Just thirty years later, it was reality.

Successful xenotransplantation would be the perfect denouement to Montgomery's career and his life. If this were a Hollywood movie, the final scene would be Montgomery wheeling back into an OR to receive his second heart, from a pig. I asked him if he would consider taking a pig heart if he were to need a second transplant. His response, which came with absolutely no hesitation, was one word. "Definitely."

* * * * *

These are my broad predictions for the next era of transplantation. It is incomplete, however, without an update on the visionaries. It's their stories that will make this all happen.

When Joe Tector returned to Miami in 2019, the place where he had completed his transplant training so many years ago, it wasn't as a conquering hero. He was appointed the director of the newly formed Xenotransplant Institute, but had a minimal role on the clinical team and was not performing transplants. To add to his misery, his wife remained in Alabama while his oldest daughter completed high school. This represented the lowest point in his professional and personal life. But with time to reflect, read, and meditate, Tector has found peace with it all. He may not be operating or running a large transplant division, and he may be temporarily separated from his beloved family, but he has accepted the reality that his life's accomplishments will be defined by the success or failure of his efforts in xenotransplantation.

In a recent interview, he was asked how he has maintained his commitment to the field of xenotransplantation for so many years, never losing his optimism despite so many setbacks. His answer seemed to address both the struggle and his peace with it. "It has possessed my entire being. I am married and I have 5 kids. But this has been soul possessing. If you see what transplant can do for an individual and for families, it is transformative. My dad was my role model and gave me so much, but having been a surgeon has been a huge driver for me. There are parts of this journey that people would tell me about, bad things, that I just didn't see. My inability to see those bad things allowed me to keep going. Ultimately, there is a scientific goal and a solution for patients here, and that's been the focus."[31] Sounds like something Winston Churchill might have said.

His company, Makana Therapeutics—which he started in 2008 under the name Xenobridge, LLC, and funded primarily with his own money— became a subsidiary of Recombinetics, a larger biotech company in the gene editing space. With a valuation of upwards of $200 million, Recombinetics has given Makana resources and leadership that will allow Tector to conduct human trials once the FDA gives him the green light. Tector continues to develop novel knockout pigs with a goal of generating animals for which humans have no natural antibodies. If anything, the recent deaths of Slayman and the two heart recipients have caused Tector to increase his efforts at generating novel pigs. He has become convinced that the currently available pigs will not be successful in trials, and the patients will require too much immunosuppression and still suffer rejection and organ loss. He has been focusing major resources on developing proprietary advanced cross-matching techniques, which may ultimately be as important as the pigs themselves. Using these techniques, Tector has identified numerous previously unrecognized natural antibodies in human samples to pig HLA molecules. This has led him to generate novel pigs with porcine HLA class I knocked out, and a class II protein eliminated as well. He is in the process of combining these pigs with his triple knockout, and expects results with these animals to be superior to anything currently available. This does deviate from his philosophy of only editing genes that evolution has deemed unnecessary, and runs the risk of altering the physiology of the organs or immune response they engender. But so far, his experiments in primates have been encouraging.

In the meantime, Tector has been breeding sibling pigs with his knockouts to generate breeding pairs to establish a herd of transgenic animals, knowing that in order to scale, cloning will be too fickle and cumbersome a technique. Tector is all in at this point. He is convinced that his strategy is the most compelling, most straightforward, most likely to succeed. His is the one company that combines mastery of gene editing and pig generation, immunology, and transplant surgery all under one roof, and in one brain. He outsources nothing. Tector's pigs may not take part in the first trials, but he is banking on long-term success with a breeding strategy that scales easily and proprietary cross-matching that may be the most advanced for all xenotransplants. He is less concerned with being first than with being successful. If he succeeds, he will enjoy both financial and reputational success, earning the moniker of pioneer. If he fails, his forty-year dream will end as a nightmare.

* * * * *

eGenesis has recently undergone a complete change in leadership, with a new CEO, CMO, and strengthened collaborations with leading academic centers. These changes led to its landmark paper on pig-to-primate outcomes and then its blockbuster pig-to-human transplants at MGH. The company remains committed to the pig with all copies of PERV disrupted, which is the background on which all their other gene edits are added. This is a big bet, as other xeno pigs have simply utilized animals that lack the PERV C genotype, which in most studies seems to be required for human cell infection *in vitro*. It remains to be seen whether the FDA will see this as a benefit, minimizing the chance of a pandemic from an endogenous retrovirus, or a risk, potentially causing an off-target effect leading to organ dysfunction, opportunistic infection, or cancer. For now, the gene targets beyond the PERV edits are fairly similar to the 10GE pig that Revivicor generated, but the gene cassettes employed by eGenesis may make future edits easier to add. In addition, eGenesis pigs are mini-swine, whereas the Revivicor pigs rely on a gene knockout to the growth hormone receptor to prevent overgrowth of organs. It's not clear whether one strategy is superior to the other.

The death of Slayman has been devastating to eGenesis and the entire transplant community, but at the same time, his normal kidney function and pathology when he died provide solace. The current success with Andrews, now thriving more than eight months removed from his xenotransplant, has electrified the xeno world. In September of 2024, the company announced the close of a $191 million series D fundraise, setting it up for future trials. The team is now approved by the FDA to conduct a twenty-patient multi-center trial once they complete their initial three patients in the protocol, which includes Andrews. The second transplant has recently been conducted. This puts them in a comparable position with United Therapeutics—or maybe even better, given the initial success with Andrews. In addition, they are approved for the clinical trial using their transgenic pigs for liver perfusion in acute liver failure, similar to those experiments conducted at the turn of the twenty-first century. It's always good to have multiple irons in the fire.

eGenesis may not be relying entirely on the FDA to move forward. In early 2024, it announced the production of genetically engineered pigs in collaboration with a company in Japan. The organ shortage in Japan is even more severe than in the United States, due to a lack of available deceased donors. The possibility of trials in Japan or potentially China, where Luhan Yang remains the CEO of Qihan Biotech, offers an alternative pathway for progress.

✳ ✳ ✳ ✳ ✳

Since her entry into the field, Martine's approach to xenotransplantation has been multipronged. Her diversified approach, with numerous strategies and multiple shots on goal, derives from her tried-and-true business tactics that have made her a pioneer and world-changer two times over. Martine's belief in the importance of gene editing and the benefits of working with world experts led her to collaborate with Venter, which in turn led to the generation of her 10GE pig that may well crack the code of xeno success. At the same time, she recognizes the challenges of getting FDA approval for this pig even with trials forthcoming, and continues to move forward with her simpler GalSafe knockout at the same time, with donor thymus thrown in. This simple Alpha Gal knockout pig already has FDA approval as a source of meat for ingestion, and it may have an easier path to approval for transplant indications. Shots on goal.

She has fruitful collaborations with Mohiuddin and Griffith at the University of Maryland and Montgomery and his team at NYU. She recently brought on board the renowned transplant surgeon Jayme Locke as the Vice President for Medical Development for xenotransplantation, solidifying her commitment to moving xenotransplantation into the clinical arena. She recently announced a collaboration with Johns Hopkins University, where the chair of surgery is Andrew Cameron, a transplant surgeon who spent his research years in David Sachs's lab. The deal included recruitment of Kaz Yamada from the Sachs/Sykes group at Columbia to Baltimore, where he will conduct kidney xenotransplants with and without the thymus, using both standard immunosuppression and tolerance protocols. The work will be supported by a $20 million commitment from United Therapeutics. Kaz recently reported impressive outcomes with the 10GE pigs using immunosuppression similar to Mohiuddin's protocol, but also some with conventional immunosuppression as well.[32] Shots on goal.

United Therapeutics recently broke ground in Christiansburg, Virginia on a facility that would have the capacity to raise and breed hundreds of transgenic pigs for pre-clinical and clinical trials. This 50,000-square-foot farm will meet the standards specified by the FDA to be designated "pathogen-free," and it is predicted to cost upwards of one hundred million dollars. It will be equipped with electric planes and drones for shipping the organs directly to the surgeons that would transplant them. It is slated to be completed imminently and will be able to deliver 125 pigs for transplant per year. Plans are also in place to build similar facilities in Texas and Minnesota.

This may sound far-fetched and futuristic, but it really isn't. Over the last decade Martine has worked with a division of United Therapeutics, Unither Bioelectronics, to develop an unmanned, carbon-neutral strategy to deliver organs across the country. The Unither Organ Delivery Systems research and development program has invested in over one thousand drones from a Chinese company, and has even successfully delivered a human lung for transplantation to the University of Toronto from another hospital in the city. As Martine said in a statement released by United Therapeutics, "We are now building drones that can fly 100 miles, and then 200 miles. Ultimately, we plan to have droned aircraft deliver lungs, hearts, and kidneys throughout all of North America." It seems worth mentioning that Martine, herself a pilot, currently holds the record for the longest flight ever accomplished in an electric helicopter—thirty-five miles.

This is just scratching the surface. In a vision reminiscent of satellites serving as canoes paddling through the sky, Martine has dreamed for years that transgenic organs would be shipped through the sky on unmanned, electric drones. In 2016, after much research, Martine made a $42 million investment in Transmedics, at the time a small company focusing on designing devices that could transport human organs on perfusion pumps to preserve their function while outside the body. This investment made United Therapeutics a significant minority owner of a company now valued in the billions. Martine cares less about the return on investment than having access to transport her bespoke pig organs to any center that might need them, arriving in prime shape and ready to be transplanted with immediate function.

If Martine has faced any obstacles in the xeno arena, it has been in transplantation of lungs, the organ that inspired her to enter the discipline in the first place. In 2006, she started a subsidiary of United Therapeutics called Lung Biotechnology, and established milestones for various prominent researchers in xenotransplantation and organ generation and repair. The xeno milestones were quickly deemed too difficult, and much of her lung funding was diverted to other efforts. After working with researchers at the University of Toronto, her team opened two lung repair centers in the United States (one in Florida with the Mayo Clinic Jacksonville and one in

North Carolina). Discarded lungs from human donors are flown to these centers, where they are placed on XVIVO perfusion pumps for resuscitation and repair and then flown back to transplant centers once they have achieved adequate function. Her team has already facilitated more than one hundred human lung transplants to date.

This strategy, while exciting, is limited by the availability of human organs. In a second, more ambitious project, researchers take pig lungs, strip them of their own cells, and repopulate the remaining scaffold with billions of human cells. A second project utilizes three-dimensional printing to make the scaffolds, which are then populated with human cells. Martine recently revealed a three-dimensional printed lung that encompassed 4,000 kilometers of pulmonary capillaries and 200 million alveoli. The printed scaffolds are showing gas exchange in animal models. Martine is optimistic that one of these strategies will solve the shortage of lungs, and predicts human trials in the five years. Shots on goal.

But what if all of this fails? While Martine is confident it won't, it may not ultimately matter. Because she is also involved in a bigger project, one that rather than focusing on replacing failing parts of a whole, will allow humans to achieve immortality during our lifetime. Martine is convinced that in a short amount of time, software will become aware, sentient. This type of prediction sounded crazy just a few years ago, but recent advances in AI have made the idea much more palatable. Martine recently published a book titled *Virtually Human*, where she "depicts a world populated by humans and their 'mindclones,' sentient digital replicas of individuals' minds, created by loading into AI video interviews, photographs, personality tests, and the entirety of their digital lives."[33] While the mindclones might exist at the same time a person was still alive, they would ultimately be immortal, existing long after the human they were cloned from was gone.

Martine conceived of United Therapeutics and became involved with xenotransplantation due to her love for Jenesis, but she has become committed to generating mindclones because of her love and devotion to Bina, the person she cannot, will not exist without. She has already made a rudimentary version of Bina in robot form (Bina48), which with current technology seems more haunting than lovable. Bina48 was recently featured in a movie, *Love Machina*, that debuted in the 2024 Sundance Film Festival. Martine and Bina have even started a "trans" religion, called Terasem, to celebrate transhumanism. It all seems a little "out of this world," but in the book *Virtually Human*, she spends many pages convincing the reader that it absolutely will happen, and then grapples with the legal standing and rights that will need to be considered for the mindclones themselves. Shots on goal.

In a recent interview in a podcast sponsored by the premiere journal *Nature*, Megan Sykes was asked what she thought were the biggest barriers that could lead to failure in xenotransplantation.[34] She was optimistic that the science would be good enough to make transgenic pig organs that would succeed, that would last long enough to be considered destination therapy and not just a bridge to a human organ. But she knew it would take time before this would be done outside of a trial, and even longer before anyone would profit from it. She had lived through the exciting years of the 1990s, when xeno seemed inevitable and companies like Novartis and Baxter were dumping money into the field. She had also lived through the 2000s, when that money rapidly disappeared and research slowed down so dramatically. Her greatest fear is that industry, a necessary partner to pay for the trials and tribulations and more trials, would lose interest, pull its money, and send xeno back to the wasteland, with success always so far in the future.

But this time is different. This time there is Martine, the visionary with billions of dollars, endless optimism, and a driving force stronger than anything else on Earth—the love for her daughter. If xeno is ever to succeed, Martine will need to keep taking shots on goal.

* * * * *

I leave you with one final prediction. I believe I will sew a pig kidney into a human in a clinical trial. I may sew a pig kidney into a human as an FDA-approved bridge while the patient waits for a human kidney. I doubt I will practice long enough to do it as a destination therapy outside of a trial. I hope I am wrong. But for those trainees that are just entering our field today, fasten your seatbelts. It's going to be a wild ride, and pig organs will be in your future. Your very near future.

Acknowledgments

I have been itching to tell the story of xeno since 2002, when the first Alpha Gal knockout pig was born. I was a general surgery resident at the University of Chicago at the time, one year removed from my fellowship in David Sachs's lab, and I had been captivated by his genius and optimism and fascinated by the experiments we were conducting. I believed then that it would change the world, and I am still convinced of that today. I proudly wear the moniker of "xeno-optimist," and I think that when xeno does finally work, it will be one of the greatest scientific advances of our lifetimes!

It has taken longer than I expected to arrive at clinical trials, but on reflection, the amount of progress that has occurred in the last two decades is mind-blowing. The intense efforts, unshakeable optimism, near-obsession, and sacrifices of those who have dedicated their lives to xeno are unmatched, and I have done my best to tell their stories. This is by no means a complete recounting of every person who has devoted his or her life to this discipline. That would be nearly impossible (and certainly unreadable). Hopefully this book does capture the genius, persistence, creativity, and accomplishments of the pioneers of our field.

First, I want to thank everyone in xeno that I was able to talk to—some for a few minutes (or a few emails), others for days and weeks on end. I connected with more than one hundred individuals who represent science, history, ethics, business, law and policy, animal rights, and perhaps most importantly, the patients. I am grateful for their honesty and insight. I considered listing each of them, but decided against it, as there are some who would rather go unmentioned. I would like to give a special thanks to a few pioneers who gave me so much of their time: Bob Montgomery, Joe Tector, and David Sachs. The three of you, along with all the other visionaries in xeno, see no hurdles too high, no criticism too crushing, no setbacks too insurmountable. In my last book about the history of transplantation and my own coming of age in the field, I spent time with the pioneers who made it happen, including Tom Starzl, Roy Calne, Paul Russell, and so many others. I wrote about their courage. It's been said that they possessed the courage to fail. They certainly had that, but I believe that so many of us in surgery (and I'm sure other professions as well) are courageous in that way. But more than that, they had the courage to succeed. They weren't afraid to push beyond all barriers, to carry on when so many of us would have given up. These people are not normal, not cut from the same cloth that most of us are. When they experienced failures, even when that meant a patient died in their hands, they persisted. They were able to persevere, because they just knew it would ultimately work out, and it would be worth it, no matter the cost. I see that in Bob and Joe, Martine, Muhammad, Bart, Tatsuo, David (all the Davids), and everyone else that will make this field happen. You have the courage to succeed. I am grateful that you chose xeno.

To my agent, Eric Lupfer—neither of my books would have seen the light of day without your support, positivity, and your ability to conceive of a path to bring my initial proposal into reality. Before I began this writing journey that started in 2016 with my first book proposal, I had no idea what an integral role an agent can play in the life of a book, from the birth of the idea to its sale to publication and beyond. You have used so much creativity in making this book happen and always stayed positive when I was feeling despair. Your calmness, confidence, vision, optimism, and decision making has been remarkable. I think a second career in surgery could work for you! I'm so glad to have you as an agent. Wait 'til you hear my next idea!

To my editors, Bob Prior and Janice Audet—Bob, thank you for selecting this proposal from the large stacks of submissions you must contend with. You gave it a chance, for which I am grateful. Thank you for reading my first draft, which I am sure was a lot longer than you were hoping. Perhaps you weren't aware that I was a Russian language and literature major in college, and had re-read *War and Peace* while working on this. Probably not the best book to model it on. Janice—thanks for taking over this project when Bob retired. I can only imagine what it is like to take on a book that you didn't acquire, but it would be nothing without your insights on structure and content. I could never have done it without you.

To my family—first to my incredible parents, Molli and Reuben. You guys are just the best. You are my first (but hopefully not only!) readers, my greatest supporters, always modeling that anything is possible. To my brothers Jon and Ben and your families—I love you guys!

And Ben—you are the GOAT! I have so enjoyed witnessing your career in the writing world, and when I finally decided to write a book you welcomed me with open arms. I don't know how you have kept it going for so long, with such optimism and confidence. You radiate so much joy in your approach to your writing and your life. You may be the most interesting person in the world. I think you have written ten books in the time it took me to write two (or maybe one). But how many transplants have you done?

To the three people and one fur ball that make my life everything that it is. Sam and Kate, I am so lucky you are my daughters! I continue to be amazed by your brilliance, joy, beauty, and humor. I love you guys and am so glad we are a family!

Gretch—I owe all my successes to you. I have never met someone like you, so brilliant, compassionate, driven. You are my moral compass. I will love you forever.

And Phoebe, we did it! Our second book together! You sat with me for all of my writing and editing, always willing to walk around the block when I was ready to take a break and clear my head. I am a bit frustrated that I have to carry you down the stairs these days, but I know you would do it for me. It also seems weird to write this for you since you can't read. But I'll give you an extra serving of the Farmer's Dog to thank you properly.

Finally, to my patients, including recipients and donors, living and deceased. I have learned so much from you and consider it the greatest privilege in my life to take part in your care. Transplantation truly is a miracle. Being part of this gift of life is intoxicating beyond words. The courage that you display is beyond belief. I consider all of us in the world of transplant part of a family, and I am thrilled and honored to be a part of it.

I have spoken to so many patients on the waitlist about the idea of accepting a pig organ and what it would mean to have that option. Universally, you have told me that the idea of this new paradigm where organs can be available when needed gives you hope. And hope is really all you have asked for. If I have any regret about the success of xeno in the future, it is that it might take away from the gift of deceased donation, the passing on of this beautiful legacy. It is the donors (living and deceased) who remind me that in this crazy world we live in, people truly want to help each other, save each other. We are all the same on the inside. Being a small part of this miraculous gift of life has maintained my belief in the good of humanity. We are all in this life together.

Notes

PREFACE

1. Rivka Galchen, "The Medical Miracle of a Pig's Heart in a Human Body," *New Yorker*, February 21, 2022, https://www.newyorker.com/magazine/2022/02/28/the-medical-miracle -of-a-pigs-heart-transplant-in-a-human-body.

2. M. Colvin et al., "OPTN/SRTR 2020 Annual Data Report: Heart," *American Journal of Transplantation* 22, Suppl 2 (2022): 350–437.

3. A .J. Kwong et al., "OPTN/SRTR 2020 Annual Data Report: Liver," *American Journal of Transplantation* 22, Suppl 2 (2022): 204–309; M. Valapour et al., "OPTN/SRTR 2020 Annual Data Report: Lung," *American Journal of Transplantation* 22, Suppl 2 (2022): 438–518.

4. K. L. Lentine et al., "OPTN/SRTR 2020 Annual Data Report: Kidney," *American Journal of Transplantation* 22, Suppl 2 (2022): 21–136.

5. Joshua D. Mezrich, *When Death Becomes Life: Notes from a Transplant Surgeon* (Harper, 2019).

CHAPTER 1

1. Abe DeAnda Jr. and Leora B. Balsam, "Historical perspectives of The American Association for Thoracic Surgery: Keith Reemtsma (1925–2000)," *Journal of Thoracic and Cardiovascular Surgery* 150, 4 (2015): 762–764.

2. Otto F. Apel and Pat Apel, *MASH: An Army Surgeon in Korea* (University Press of Kentucky: 1998).

3. Abe DeAnda Jr. and Leora B. Balsam, "Historical perspectives of The American Association for Thoracic Surgery: Keith Reemtsma (1925–2000)," *Journal of Thoracic and Cardiovascular Surgery* 150, 4 (2015): 762–764.

4. David Hamilton, *A History of Organ Transplantation: Ancient Legends to Modern Practice* (University of Pittsburgh Press: 2012).

5. "Doctors Transplant Kidneys of Monkey to Young Woman," *Dallas Morning News*, 1963.

6. Mark A. Hardy, *Xenograft 25: proceedings of the International Congress, Xenograft 25, held at Arden House, Harriman, New York, 11–13 November 1988* (Excerpta Medicine, 1989).

7. J. Osmundsen, "2 Monkey Kidneys Transplanted to Woman in Pioneer Operation," *New York Times*, 1963.

8. Keith Reemtsma et al., "Renal Heterotransplantation in Man," *Annals of Surgery* 160, no. 3 (1964): 384–410.

9. *History of Transplantation: Thirty-Five Recollections*, ed. Paul Terasaki (UCLA Immunogenetics Center: 1991).

10. Keith Reemtsma, "Reversal of Early Graft Rejection after Renal Heterotransplantation in Man," *JAMA* 187, no.10 (1964): 691–696.

11. "Man Regains Health with Chimp Kidney," *Los Angeles Times*, 1963.

12. N. Taylor, "Heart to Heart: Can a Chimp Transplant Save Human Life?" *New York Magazine*, 1987.

13. J. Russel Elkington, "Moral Problems in the Use of Borrowed Organs, Artificial and Transplanted," *Annals of Internal Medicine* 60, no. 2 (1965): 309–313, https://repository.library .georgetown.edu/handle/10822/762416.

14. Mark A. Hardy, *Xenograft 25: proceedings of the International Congress, Xenograft 25, held at Arden House, Harriman, New York, 11–13 November 1988* (Excerpta Medicine, 1989).

15. David Cooper, *Open Heart: The Radical Surgeons Who Revolutionized Medicine* (Kaplan Publishing: 2010).

16. Thomas Starzl et al., "Renal Heterotransplantation from Baboon to Man: Experience with 6 Cases," *Transplantation* 2 (1964): 752–776.

17. Mark A. Hardy, *Xenograft 25: proceedings of the International Congress, Xenograft 25, held at Arden House, Harriman, New York, 11–13 November 1988* (Excerpta Medicine, 1989).

18. Geoffrey R. Giles, "Clinical Heterotransplantation of the Liver," *Transplant Proceedings* 2, no. 4 (1970): 506–512.

19. David Cooper, "Early Clinical Xenotransplantation Experiences-An Interview with Thomas E. Starzl, MD, PhD," *Xenotransplantation* 24, no. 2 (2017).

CHAPTER 2

1. *Stephanie's Heart: The Story of Baby Fae*, dir. Michael Wilcott, 1 hour, Loma Linda University Health, December 23, 2015, https://www.youtube.com/watch?v=sQbJ0WP-wn4.

2. Leonard L. Bailey, "Remembering Baby Fae," Loma Linda University Adventist Health Sciences Center (2007).

3. Leonard L. Bailey, "Another Look at Cardiac Xenotransplantation," *Journal of Cardiothoracic Surgery* 5, no. 3 (1990): 210–218; Leonard L. Bailey and S. R. Gundry, "Survival Following

Orthotopic Cardiac Xenotransplantation Between Juvenile Baboon Recipients and Concordant and Discordant Donor Species: Foundation for Clinical Trials," *World Journal of Surgery* 21, no. 9 (1997): 943–950.

4.   Leonard L. Bailey, "Remembering Baby Fae," Loma Linda University Adventist Health Sciences Center (2007).

5.   Leonard L. Bailey, "Remembering Baby Fae," Loma Linda University Adventist Health Sciences Center (2007).

6.   *Stephanie's Heart: The Story of Baby Fae*, dir. Michael Wilcott, 1 hour, Loma Linda University Health, December 23, 2015, https://www.youtube.com/watch?v=sQbJ0WP-wn4.

7.   Leonard L. Bailey, "Remembering Baby Fae," Loma Linda University Adventist Health Sciences Center (2007).

8.   *Stephanie's Heart: The Story of Baby Fae*, dir. Michael Wilcott, 1 hour, Loma Linda University Health, December 23, 2015, https://www.youtube.com/watch?v=sQbJ0WP-wn4.

9.   Leonard L. Bailey, "Remembering Baby Fae," Loma Linda University Adventist Health Sciences Center (2007).

10.   Tony Stark, *Knife to the Heart: Story of Transplant Surgery* (Macmillan, 1996).

11.   Stark, *Knife to the Heart*.

12.   Leo Gutkind, *Many Sleepless Nights: The World of Organ Transplantation* (W. W. Norton & Co., 1988).

13.   *Stephanie's Heart: The Story of Baby Fae*, dir. Michael Wilcott, 1 hour, Loma Linda University Health, December 23, 2015, https://www.youtube.com/watch?v=sQbJ0WP-wn4.

14.   Leonard L. Bailey et al., "Baboon-to-Human Cardiac Xenotransplantation in a Neonate," *JAMA* 254, no. 23 (1985): 3321–3329.

15.   *Stephanie's Heart*, dir. Michael Wilcott.

16.   *Stephanie's Heart*, dir. Michael Wilcott.

17.   L. L. Bailey, "Remembering Baby Fae," 2007; Larry Kidder, "Stephanie's Heart: The Story of Baby Fae," Loma Linda University Health, September 8, 2016, https://web.archive.org/web/20200104034647/https://news.llu.edu/patient-care/stephanie-s-heart-story-of-baby-fae.

18.   Stark, *Knife to the Heart*.

19.   *Stephanie's Heart*, dir. Michael Wilcott.

20.   Bailey, "Remembering Baby Fae"; Kidder, "Stephanie's Heart."

21.   Bailey, "Remembering Baby Fae."

22.   Mark A. Hardy, *Xenograft 25: proceedings of the International Congress, Xenograft 25, held at Arden House, Harriman, New York, 11–13 November 1988* (Excerpta Medicine, 1989).

CHAPTER 3

1. *Recollections of Pioneers in Xenotransplantation Research*, ed. David Cooper (Nova Science Pub., 2018).

2. R. J. Perper and J. S. Najarian, "Experimental Renal Heterotransplantation. I. In widely divergent species." *Transplantation* 4, no. 4 (1966): 377–388.

3. David Cooper et al., "Pig Liver Xenotransplantation: A Review of Progress Toward the Clinic," *Transplantation* 100, no. 10 (2016): 2039–2047.

4. *Recollections of Pioneers in Xenotransplantation Research*, ed. David Cooper (Nova Science Pub., 2018); G. Wayne Miller, *The Xeno Chronicles: Two Years on the Frontier of Medicine Inside Harvard's Transplant Research Lab* (PublicAffairs, 2005).

5. Uri Galili, "Discovery of the Natural Anti-Gal Antibody and its Past and Future Relevance to Medicine," *Xenotransplantation* 20, no. 3(2013): 138–147.

6. Uri Galili et al., "A Unique Natural Human IgG Antibody with Anti-Alpha-Galactosyl Specificity," *Journal of Experimental Medicine* 160, no. 5 (1984): 1519–1531; Uri Galili, "Anti-Gal: An Abundant Human Natural Antibody of Multiple Pathogeneses and Clinical Benefits," *Immunology* 140, no. 1 (2013): 1–11.

7. Tony Stark, *Knife to the Heart: Story of Transplant Surgery* (Macmillan, 1996).

8. Peter F. Zipfel and Christine Skerka, "From Magic Bullets to Modern Therapeutics: Paul Ehrlich, the German Immunobiologist and Physician Coined the Term 'Complement.'" *Molecular Immunology* 150 (2022): 90–98.

9. Juan Carlos Varela and Stephen Tomlinson, "Complement: An Overview for the Clinician," *Hematology/Oncology Clinics of North America* 29, no. 3 (2015): 409–427.

10. H. Gewurz et al., "Effect of cobra venom-induced inhibition of complement activity on allograft and xenograft rejection reactions," *Transplantation* 5, no. 5 (1967): 1296–1303.

11. E. Kemp et al., "Delayed Rejection of Rabbit Kidneys Transplanted into Baby Pigs," *Transplant Proceedings* 19, no. 1 (1987): 1143–1144.

12. Stark, *Knife to the Heart*; Jenny Bryan and John Clare, *Organ Farm* (Carlton Books Limited, 2001).

13. *Recollections of Pioneers in Xenotransplantation Research*, ed. David Cooper (Nova Science Pub., 2018); Emanuele Cozzi et al., "David J. G. White, PhD, FRCPath," *Xenotransplantation* 24, no. 5 (2017).

14. Mauricio Rocha-Martins et al., "From Gene Targeting to Genome Editing: Transgenic Animals Applications and Beyond," *Anais da Academia Brasileira de* Ciências 87, no. 2 (2015): 1323–1348; Dmitriy Myelnikov, "Tinkering with Genes and Embryos: The Multiple Invention of Transgenic Mice c. 1980." *History and Technology* 35, no. 4 (2019): 425–452.

15. David Cooper and Robert Lanza, *XENO: The Promise of Transplanting Animal Organs into Humans* (Oxford University Press, 2000).

16. G. Wayne Miller, *The Xeno Chronicles: Two Years on the Frontier of Medicine Inside Harvard's Transplant Research Lab* (PublicAffairs, 2005).

17. Miller, *The Xeno Chronicles.*

18. Miller.

19. R. E. Billingham et al., "Actively Acquired Tolerance of Foreign Cells," *Nature* 172, 4379 (1953): 603–606.

20. David H. Sachs, "The Medawar Prize Acceptance Speech 2014," *Transplantation* 99, no. 2 (2015): 254–257.

21. David H. Sachs and James L. Cone, "A Mouse B-cell Alloantigen Determined by Gene(s) Linked to the Major Histocompatibility Complex," *Journal of Experimental Medicine* 138, no. 6 (1973): 1289–1304.

22. Jacques Neefjes et al., "Towards a Systems Understanding of MHC Class I and MHC Class II Antigen Presentation," *Nature Reviews Immunolology* 11, no. 12 (2011): 823–836.

23. David H. Sachs et al., "Induction of Tolerance Through Mixed Chimerism," *CSH Perspectives in Medicine* 4, no. 1 (2014); David H. Sachs, "Transplantation Tolerance Through Mixed Chimerism: From Allo to Xeno," *Xenotransplantation* 25, no. 3 (2018).

24. K. Yamada, "Influence of the Thymus on Transplantation Tolerance in Miniature Swine," *Transplantation Proceedings* 29 no. 1–2 (1997): 1076.

25. Brahma Kumar, "Human T Cell Development, Localization, and Function Throughout Life," *Immunity* 48, no. 2 (2018): 202–213.

CHAPTER 4

1. *Recollections of Pioneers in Xenotransplantation Research*, ed. David Cooper (Nova Science Pub., 2018).

2. *PBS Frontline*, "Organ Farm," March 27, 2001, https://www.pbs.org/wgbh/pages/frontline/shows/organfarm/.

3. Emanuele Cozzi and David J. G. White, "The Generation of Transgenic Pigs as Potential Organ Donors for Humans," *Nature Medicine* 1, no. 9 (1995): 964–966.

4. *Recollections of Pioneers*, ed. David Cooper.

5. Henk-Jan Schuurman et al., "Incidence of Hyperacute Rejection in Pig-to-Primate Transplantation Using Organs From hDAF-Transgenic Donors," *Transplantation* 73, no. 7 (2002): 1146–1151.

6. Jeremy Laurance, "Could These Priceless Pigs Help Save Thousands of Human Lives Each Year?" *Independent*, August 20, 1999, https://www.independent.co.uk/news/could-these-priceless-pigs-help-save-thousands-of-human-lives-each-year-1113725.html.

7. A. Zaidi et al., "Life-Supporting Pig-to-Primate Renal Xenotransplantation Using Genetically Modified Donors," *Transplantation* 65, no. 12 (1998): 1584–1590.

8. Emanuele Cozzi et al., "Long-Term Survival of Nonhuman Primates Receiving Life-Supporting Transgenic Porcine Kidney Xenografts," *Transplantation* 70, no. 1 (2000): 15–21.

9. *PBS Frontline*, "Organ Farm."

10. *PBS Frontline*, "Organ Farm."

11. *New Scientist*, "In Brief: Foreign Organs," April 27, 1996, https://www.newscientist.com/article/mg15020271-900-in-brief-foreign-organs/.

12. Sheryl Gay Stolberg, "Could This Pig Save Your Life?" *New York Times Magazine*, October 3, 1999, https://www.nytimes.com/1999/10/03/magazine/could-this-pig-save-your-life.html.

13. R. S. Chari et al., "Brief report: treatment of hepatic failure with ex vivo pig-liver perfusion followed by liver transplantation," *New England Journal of Medicine* 331, no. 4 (1994): 234–237.

14. "Could This Pig Save Your Life?" Stolberg; Jenny Bryan and John Clare, *Organ Farm* (Carlton Books Limited, 2001).

15. G. Wayne Miller, *The Xeno Chronicles: Two Years on the Frontier of Medicine Inside Harvard's Transplant Research Lab* (PublicAffairs, 2005).

16. Kazuhiko Yamada et al., "Thymic transplantation in miniature swine. I. Development and function of the 'thymokidney.'" *Transplantation* 68, no. 11 (1999): 1684–1692.

17. Karl Illmensee and Peter C. Hoppe, "Nuclear Transplantation in Mus Musculus: Developmental Potential of Nuclei from Preimplantation Embryos," *Cell* 23, no. 1 (1981): 9–18.

18. Steen M. Willadsen and R. A. Godke, "A Simple Procedure for the Production of Identical Sheep Twins," *Veterinary Record* 114, no. 10 (1984): 240–243; Steen M. Willadsen, "Nuclear Transplantation in Sheep Embryos," *Nature* 320 (1986): 63–65.

19. Randall S. Prather et al., "Nuclear Transplantation in the Bovine Embryo: Assessment of Donor Nuclei and Recipient Oocyte," *Biology of Reproduction* 37, no. 4 (1987): 859–866.

20. K. H. Campbell, "Sheep Cloned by Nuclear Transfer from a Cultured Cell Line," *Nature* 380 (1996): 64–66.

21. I. Wilmut et al., "Viable Offspring Derived from Fetal and Adult Mammalian Cells," *Nature* 385 (1997): 810–813.

22. Angelika E. Schnieke et al., "Human Factor IX Transgenic Sheep Produced by Transfer of Nuclei from Transfected Fetal Fibroblasts," *Science* 278 (1997): 2130–2133.

23. Mauricio Rocha-Martins et al., "From Gene Targeting to Genome Editing: Transgenic Animals Applications and Beyond," *Anais da Academia Brasileira de* Ciências 87, no. 2 (2015): 1323–1348

24. National Human Genome Research Institute, "Homologous Recombination," *Talking Glossary of Genomic and Genetic Terms*, https://www.genome.gov/genetics-glossary.

25. Oliver Smithies et al., "Insertion of DNA Sequences into the Human Chromosomal Beta-Globin Locus by Homologous Recombination," *Nature* 317 (1985): 230–234.

26. Gina Kolata, "Scientist Reports First Cloning Ever of Adult Mammal," *New York Times*, February 23, 1997, https://www.nytimes.com/1997/02/23/us/scientist-reports-first-cloning -ever-of-adult-mammal.html.

27. Marjorie Miller, "5 pigs Cloned; Transplants to Humans Touted," *Los Angeles Times*, March 15, 2000.

28. Miller, *The Xeno Chronicles*.

29. John C. LaMattina, "Vascularized thymic lobe transplantation in miniature swine: I. Vascularized thymic lobe allografts support thymopoiesis," *Transplantation* 73, no. 5 (2002): 826–831.

30. Liangxue Lai et al., "Production of Apha-1,3-galactosyltransferase Knockout Pigs by Nuclear Transfer Cloning," *Science* 295 (2002): 1089–1092.

31. James Meek, "Cloned Pigs Give Vital Boost to Future of Transplants," *The Guardian*, January 3, 2002.

32. T. F. Library, "World's First Double Gene 'Knock-out' Could Be Major Breakthrough in Success of Xenotransplantation."

CHAPTER 5

1. Brigid Brophy, "The Rights of Animals," *The Sunday Times*, 1965.

2. *Animals, Men and Morals: An Inquiry into the Maltreatment of Non-humans*, ed. Stanley Godlovitch, Roslind Godlovitch, and John Harris (Grove Press, 1971).

3. Peter Singer, *Animal Liberation: A New Ethics for our Treatment of Animals*. (HarperCollins, 1975).

4. Jenny Bryan and John Clare, *Organ Farm* (Carlton Books Limited, 2001).

5. Bryan and Claire, *Organ Farm*.

6. Mark Townsend, "Exposed: Secrets of the Animal Organ Lab," *The Guardian*, April 20, 2003, https://www.theguardian.com/uk/2003/apr/20/health.businessofresearch#:~:text=The%20 papers%20reveal%20attempts%20to,regulations%20were%20not%20enforced%20 properly.

7. Bryan and Claire, *Organ Farm*.

8. G. Wayne Miller, *The Xeno Chronicles: Two Years on the Frontier of Medicine Inside Harvard's Transplant Research Lab* (PublicAffairs, 2005).

9. R. A. Weiss and L. N. Payne, "The Heritable Nature of the Factor in Chicken Cells Which Acts as a Helper Virus for Rous Sarcoma Virus," *Virology* 45, no. 2 (1971): 508–515.

10. A. G. Dalgleish et al., "The CD4 (T4) Antigen is an Essential Component of the Receptor for the AIDS Retrovirus," *Nature* 312 (1984): 763–767.

11. *RNA Tumor Viruses*, ed. Robin Weiss and A. Bernstein (Cold Spring Harbor Lab Press, 1984).

12. Edward B. Chuong, "The Placenta Goes Viral: Retroviruses Control Gene Expression in Pregnancy," *PLOS Biology* 16, no. 10 (2018).

13. Robin A. Weiss, "Circe, Cassandra, and the Trojan Pigs: Xenotransplantation," *Proceedings of the American Philosophical Society* 148, no. 3 (2004): 281–295.

14. J. M. Coffin, "Endogenous Viruses," in *Molecular Biology of Tumor Viruses*, 2nd ed., vol. 10: *RNA Tumor Viruses*, ed. R. Weiss et al., 1109–1204 (Cold Spring Harbor Laboratory, 1982).

15. Jonathan P. Stoye and John M. Coffin, "The Dangers of Xenotransplantation." *Nature Medicine* 1, no. 11 (1995): 1100.

16. Clive Patience et al., "Infection of Human Cells by an Endogenous Retrovirus of Pigs," *Nature Medicine* 3, no. 3 (1997): 282–286.

17. Jon Allan, "Silk Purse or Sow's Ear," *Nature Medicine* 3, no. 3 (1997): 275–276.

18. Walid Heneine et al., "No Evidence of Infection with Porcine Endogenous Retrovirus in Recipients of Porcine Islet-Cell Xenografts," *Lancet* 352, no. 9129 (1998): 695–699; Clive Patience, "No Evidence of Pig DNA or Retroviral Infection in Patients with Short-Term Extracorporeal Connection to Pig Kidneys," *Lancet* 352, no. 9129 (1998): 699–701; Khazal Paradis et al., "Search for Cross-Species Transmission of Porcine Endogenous Retrovirus in Patients Treated with Living Pig Tissue. The XEN 111 Study Group." *Science* 285, no. 5431 (1999): 1236–1241.

19. Weiss, "Circe, Cassandra, and the Trojan Pigs."

20. F. H. Bach and M. L. Bach, "Mixed Leukocyte Cultures in Transplantation Immunology," *Transplantation Proceedings* 3, no. 1 (1971): 942–948.

21. Fritz H. Bach et al., "Bone-Marrow Transplantation in a Patient with the Wiskott-Aldrich Syndrome," *Lancet* 2, no. 7583 (1968): 1364–1366.

22. Fritz H. Bach et al., "Uncertainty in Xenotransplantation: Individual Benefit Versus Collective Risk," *Nature Medicine* 4, no. 2 (1998): 141–144.

23. David H. Sachs et al., "Xenotransplantation—Caution, But No Moratorium," *Nature Medicine* 4, no. 4 (1998): 372–373.

24. Robin A. Weiss, "Certain Promise and Uncertain Peril. The Debate on Xenotransplantation," *EMBO Reports* 1, no. 1 (2000): 2–4.

25. Weiss, "Circe, Cassandra, and the Trojan Pigs."

26. Kazuhiko Yamada et al., "Marked Prolongation of Porcine Renal Xenograft Survival in Baboons Through the Use of Alpha1,3-Galactosyltransferase Gene-Knockout Donors and the Cotransplantation of Vascularized Thymic Tissue," *Nature Medicine* 11, no. 1 (2005): 32–34.

27. Kenji Kuwaki et al., "Heart Transplantation in Baboons Using Alpha1,3-Galactosyltransferase Gene-Knockout Pigs as Donors: Initial Experience," *Nature Medicine* 11, no. 1 (2005): 29–31.

28. Miller, *The Xeno Chronicles*.

29. Miller, *The Xeno Chronicles*.

30. Miller, *The Xeno Chronicles*.

31. Franklin Hoke, "As Cross-Species Transplantation Forges Ahead, Some Researchers Call for Caution," *The Scientist*, 1995, https://www.the-scientist.com/as-cross-species-transplantation-forges-ahead-some-researchers-call-for-caution-58394.

32. Laurel L. Yasko et al., "Committee for Oversight of Research Involving the Dead (CORID): Insights from The First Year," *Cambridge Quarterly of Healthcare Ethics* 13, no. 4 (2004): 327–337.

33. "Medical Research at the Edge of Death Presents Quandary," *Baltimore Sun*, February 2, 2003.

CHAPTER 6

1. "Martine Rothblatt—A Masterclass on Asking Better Questions and Peering into the Future," *The Tim Ferriss Show*, December 16, 2020.

2. Neely Tucker, "Martine Rothblatt: She founded SiriusXM, a religion and a biotech. For starters," *The Washington Post*, December 12, 2014.

3. Rebecca Harrington, "How A Millionaire Saved Her Daughter's Life—And Tens of Thousands of Others in The Process," *Business Insider*, May 5, 2016.

4. Lisa Miller, "The Trans-Everything CEO," *New York Magazine*, September 7, 2014.

5. "Martine Rothblatt," *The Tim Ferriss Show*.

6. "Martine Rothblatt," *The Tim Ferriss Show*.

7. Miller, "The Trans-Everything CEO."

8. M. Rothblatt, *make it*. K. Little, MSNBC.

9. Martine Rothblatt, "My Daughter, My Wife, Our Robot, And the Quest for Immortality," *TED*, March 2015.

10. Rothblatt, *make it*. K. Little, MSNBC.

11. Miller, "The Trans-Everything CEO."

12. Martine Rothblatt, *The Apartheid of Sex: A Manifesto on The Freedom of Gender* (Crown Publishers: 1995)

13. Rothblatt, *Apartheid of Sex*.

14. Miller, "The Trans-Everything CEO."

15. Miller, "The Trans-Everything CEO."

16. Miller, "The Trans-Everything CEO."

17. "Martine Rothblatt," *The Tim Ferriss Show*.

18. Tom Clynes, "20 Americans Die Each Day Waiting for Organ. Can Pigs Save Them?" *New York Times Magazine*, November 14, 2018.

19. T. Greidanus, dir., *Burden of Genius*, 2017, 1:28.

20. Rajat M. Gupta and Kiran Musunuru, "Expanding the Genetic Editing Tool Kit: ZFNs, TALENs, and CRISPR-Cas9," *Journal of Clinical Investigation* 124, no. 10 (2014): 4154–4161.

21. Aaron Klug, "The Discovery of Zinc Fingers and Their Development for Practical Applications in Gene Regulation and Genome Manipulation," *Annual Review of Biochemistry* 79 (2010): 1–21.

22. Srinivasan Chandrasegaran and Dana Carroll, "Origins of Programmable Nucleases for Genome Engineering." *Journal of Molecular Biology* 428, no. 5 (2016): 963–989.

23. Sanjeev Waghmare et al., "Gene Targeting and Cloning in Pigs Using Fetal Liver Derived Cells," *Journal of Surgical Research* 171, no. 2 (2011): e223–229.

24. Ping Li et al., "Biallelic Knockout of The Alpha-1,3 Galactosyltransferase Gene in Porcine Liver-Derived Cells Using Zinc Finger Nucleases," *Journal of Surgical Research* 181, no. 1 (2013): e39–45.

25. Andrew J. Lutz et al., "Double Knockout Pigs Deficient In N-Glycolylneuraminic Acid and Galactose Alpha-1,3-Galactose Reduce the Humoral Barrier to Xenotransplantation," *Xenotransplantation* 20, 1 (2013): 27–35.

26. C. Burlak et al., "Reduced Binding of Human Antibodies to Cells from GGTA1/CMAH KO Pigs," *American Journal of Transplantation* 14, no. 8 (2014): 1895–1900.

27. Jose Estrada et al., "Evaluation of Human and Non-Human Primate Antibody Binding to Pig Cells Lacking GGTA1/CMAH/beta4GalNT2 genes," *Xenotransplantation* 22, 3 (2015): 194–202.

28. Burlak et al., "Reduced Binding of Human Antibodies."

29. Le Cong et al., "Multiplex Genome Engineering Using CRISPR/Cas Systems," *Science* 339, no. 6121 (2013): 819–823.

30. Prashant Mali et al., "RNA-Guided Human Genome Engineering Via Cas9," *Science* 339, no. 6121 (2013): 823–826.

31. Rajat M. Gupta and Kiran Musunuru, "Expanding the Genetic Editing Tool Kit: ZFNs, TALENs, and CRISPR-Cas9," *Journal of Clinical Investigation* 124, no. 10 (2014): 4154–4161.

32. Jennifer A. Doudna and Emmanuelle Charpentier, "Genome Editing. The new Frontier of Genome Engineering with CRISPR-Cas9," *Science* 346, no. 6213 (2014).

33. Ping Li et al., "Efficient Generation of Genetically Distinct Pigs in a Single Pregnancy Using Multiplexed Single-Guide RNA and Carbohydrate Selection," *Xenotransplantation* 22, no. 1 (2015): 20–31.

34. Personal communication.

35. Personal communication.

36. Martine Rothblatt, *Your Life or Mine: How Geoethics Can Resolve the Conflict Between Public and Private Interests in Xenotransplantation* (Ashgate Publishing: 2003).

37. Martin Jinek et al., "A Programmable Dual-RNA-Guided DNA Endonuclease in Adaptive Bacterial Immunity," *Science* 337, no. 6096 (2012): 816–821; Martin Jinek et al., "RNA-Programmed Genome Editing in Human Cells," *Elife* 2: e00471 (2013).

38. Le Cong et al., "Multiplex Genome Engineering Using CRISPR/Cas Systems," *Science* 339, no. 6121 (2013): 819–823.

39. Mali, "RNA-guided human genome engineering."

40. Luhan Yang et al., "Genome-wide Inactivation of Porcine Endogenous Retroviruses (PERVs)," *Science* 350, no. 6264 (2015): 1101–1104.

41. Robert D. Fleischmann et al., "Whole-Genome Random Sequencing and Assembly of Haemophilus Influenzae Rd." *Science* 269, no. 5223 (1995): 496–512.

42. J. Craig Venter et al., "The Sequence of the Human Genome," *Science* 291, no. 5507 (2001): 1304–1351.

43. Daniel G. Gibson et al., "Creation of a Bacterial Cell Controlled by a Chemically Synthesized Genome," *Science* 329, no. 5987 (2010): 52–56.

44. United Therapeutics, "Press Release: Synthetic Genomics Inc. Signs Collaborative Research and Development Agreement with Lung Biotechnology Inc., a Subsidiary of United Therapeutics Corporation, to Develop Humanized Pig Organs to Revolutionize Transplantation Field," May 6, 2014, https://ir.unither.com/press-releases/2014/05-06-2014-095453185.

45. Dong Niu et al., "Inactivation of Porcine Endogenous Retrovirus in Pigs Using CRISPR-Cas9," *Science* 357, no. 6357 (2017): 1303–1307.

46. Karen Weintraub, "Gene-Editing Success Brings Pig-to-Human Transplants Closer to Reality," *Scientific American*, August 10, 2017, https://www.scientificamerican.com/article/gene-editing-success-brings-pig-to-human-transplants-closer-to-reality/.

CHAPTER 7

1. Rimal Farrukh, "The Muslim Doctor Behind the First Cocaine-laced Pig-to-Human Heart Transplant," *Vice*, January 21, 2022.

2. Farrukh, "The Muslim Doctor Behind the First Cocaine-laced Pig-to-Human Heart Transplant."

3. Allan D. Kirk et al., "Treatment with Humanized Monoclonal Antibody Against CD154 Prevents Acute Renal Allograft Rejection in Nonhuman Primates," *Nature Medicine* 5, no. 6 (1999): 686–693.

4. Rivka Galchen, "The Medical Miracle of a Pig's Heart in a Human Body," *New Yorker*, February 21, 2022, https://www.newyorker.com/magazine/2022/02/28/the-medical-miracle -of-a-pigs-heart-transplant-in-a-human-body.

5. Muhammad Mohiuddin et al., "B-Cell Depletion Extends the Survival of GTKO.hCD46Tg Pig Heart Xenografts in Baboons for Up to 8 Months," *American Journal of Transplantation* 12, no. 3 (2012): 763–771.

6. Muhammad Mohiuddin et al., "One-year Heterotopic Cardiac Xenograft Survival in a Pig to Baboon Model," *American Journal of Transplantation* 14, no. 2 (2014): 488–489.

7. Muhammad Mohiuddin et al., "Chimeric 2C10R4 Anti-CD40 Antibody Therapy is Critical for Long-Term Survival of GTKO.hCD46.hTBM Pig-to-Primate Cardiac Xenograft," *Nature Communications* 7 (2016).

8. Personal communication.

9. Jose L. Estrada et al., "Evaluation of Human and Non-Human Primate Antibody Binding to Pig Cells Lacking GGTA1/CMAH/beta4GalNT2 Genes." *Xenotransplantation* 22, no. 3 (2015): 194–202.

10. Personal communication.

11. Personal communication.

12. Personal communication.

13. Karen Weintraub, "Meet the Pigs That Could Solve the Human Organ Transplant Crisis," *MIT Technology Review*, November 1, 2019.

14. Ulrike Brandl et al., "Transgenic Animals in Experimental Xenotransplantation Models: Orthotopic Heart Transplantation in the Pig-to-Baboon Model," *Transplantation Proceedings* 39, no. 2 (2007): 577–578.

15. Matthias Langin et al., "Consistent Success in Life-Supporting Porcine Cardiac Xenotransplantation," *Nature* 564, no. 7736 (2018): 430–433.

16. Weintraub, "Meet the Pigs."

17. Arne Hinrichs et al., "Growth Hormone Receptor Knockout to Reduce the Size of Donor Pigs for Preclinical Xenotransplantation Studies," *Xenotransplantation* 28, no. 2 (2021): e12664.

18. Steven C. Kim et al., "Long-term Survival of Pig-to-Rhesus Macaque Renal Xenografts is Dependent on CD4 T Cell Depletion," *American Journal of Transplantation* 19, no. 8 (2019): 2174–2185.

19. Andrew B. Adams et al., "Xenoantigen Deletion and Chemical Immunosuppression Can Prolong Renal Xenograft Survival," *Annals of Surgery* 268, no. 4 (2018): 564–573.

20. Adams et al., "Xenoantigen Deletion and Chemical Immunosuppression."

21. Andrew B. Adams et al., "Anti-C5 Antibody Tesidolumab Reduces Early Antibody-mediated Rejection and Prolongs Survival in Renal Xenotransplantation," *Annals of Surgery* 274, no. 3 (2021): 473–480.

22. Thomas J. McFeeley, "Change of Heart: Transplant Pioneer Uses Experience as a Patient to Develop Landmark Innovation," *American College of Surgeons Bulletin*, September 1, 2022.

23. McFeeley, "Change of Heart."

24. "Episode 8: Dr. Robert Montgomery on Resilience," *The Sett*, Joshua D. Mezrich, April 3, 2021.

25. Mezrich, "Episode 8."

26. Mezrich, "Episode 8."

27. Mezrich, "Episode 8."

28. Dorry L. Segev et al., "Kidney Paired Donation and Optimizing the Use of Live Donor Organs," *JAMA* 293, no. 15 (2005): 1883–1890.

29. Michael A. Rees et al., "A Nonsimultaneous, Extended, Altruistic-Donor Chain," *New England Journal of Medicine* 360, no. 11 (2009): 1096–1101.

30. Robert A. Montgomery et al., "Desensitization in HLA-Incompatible Kidney Recipients and Survival," *New England Journal of Medicine* 365, no. 4 (2011): 318–326.

31. Mezrich, "Episode 8."

32. Mezrich, "Episode 8."

33. Mezrich, "Episode 8."

34. Mezrich, "Episode 8."

35. McFeeley, "Change of Heart."

36. McFeeley, "Change of Heart."

CHAPTER 8

1. Roni Caryn Rabin, "In a First, Surgeons Attached a Pig Kidney to a Human, and It Worked." *New York Times*, October 19, 2021.

2. Rabin, "In a First, Surgeons Attached a Pig Kidney to a Human."

3. Rabin, "In a First, Surgeons Attached a Pig Kidney to a Human."

4. Paige M. Porrett, "First Clinical-Grade Porcine Kidney Xenotransplant Using a Human Decedent Model," *American Journal of Transplantation* 22, no. 4 (2022): 1037–1053.

5. Robert A. Montgomery, "Results of Two Cases of Pig-to-Human Kidney Xenotransplantation," *New England Journal of Medicine* 386, 20 (2022): 1889–1898.

6. Nader Moazami et al., "Pig-To-Human Heart Xenotransplantation in Two Recently Deceased Human Recipients," *Nature Medicine* 29, no.8 (2023): 1989–1997.

7. Rabin, "In a First, Surgeons Attached a Pig Kidney to a Human."

8. Rivka Galchen, "The Medical Miracle of a Pig's Heart in a Human Body," *New Yorker*, February 21, 2022, https://www.newyorker.com/magazine/2022/02/28/the-medical-miracle-of-a-pigs-heart-transplant-in-a-human-body.

9. Laura DiChiacchio et al., "Early Experience with Preclinical Perioperative Cardiac Xenograft Dysfunction in a Single Program," *The Annals of Thoracic Surgery* 109, no. 5 (2020): 1357–1361.

10. Rimal Farrukh, "The Muslim Doctor Behind the First Cocaine-laced Pig-to-Human Heart Transplant," *Vice*, January 21, 2022.

11. Muhammad Mohiuddin, "Progressive Genetic Modifications of Porcine Cardiac Xenografts Extend Survival To 9 Months," *Xenotransplantation* 29, no. 3 (2022).

12. David K. Cooper, "Report of the Xenotransplantation Advisory Committee of the International Society for Heart and Lung Transplantation: The Present Status of Xenotransplantation and its Potential Role in the Treatment of End-Stage Cardiac and Pulmonary Diseases," *The Journal of Heart and Lung Transplantation* 19, no. 12 (2000): 1125–1165.

13. Galchen, "The Medical Miracle of a Pig's Heart in a Human Body."

14. Rabin, "In a First, Surgeons Attached a Pig Kidney to a Human."

15. Bartley P. Griffith, "Genetically Modified Porcine-to-Human Cardiac Xenotransplantation," *New England Journal of Medicine* 387, no. 1 (2022): 35–44.

16. University of Maryland School of Medicine, "In Memoriam: David Bennett, Sr.," March 9, 2022, https://www.medschool.umaryland.edu/news/2022/in-memoriam-david-bennett -sr.html.

17. Carla K. Johnson, "In 1st, US Surgeons Transplant Pig Heart into Human Patient," *Associated Press*, January 10, 2022, https://apnews.com/article/pig-heart-transplant-6651614cb9 d73bada8eea2ecb6449aef.

18. Lauran Neergaard and Carla K. Johnson, "A Man Who Got The 1st Pig Heart Transplant Dies After 2 Months," *Associated Press*, March 9, 2022, https://apnews.com/article/ pig-heart-transplant-patient-dies-bc3b304de3c8d3bf3acbb3c221960.

19. University of Maryland School of Medicine, "In Memoriam: Lawrence Faucette," October 31, 2023, https://www.medschool.umaryland.edu/news/2023/in-memoriam-lawrence -faucette.html.

20. Galchen, "The Medical Miracle of a Pig's Heart in a Human Body."

21. Lauran Neergaard and Shelby Lum, "Pig Kidney Works a Record 2 Months in Donated Body, Raising Hope for Animal-Human Transplants," *Associated Press*, September 14, 2023.

22. Roni Caryn Rabin, "Surgeons Transplant Pig Kidney into a Patient, a Medical Milestone," *New York Times*, March 21, 2024.

23. Ranjith P. Anand, "Design and Testing of a Humanized Porcine Donor for Xenotransplantation," *Nature* 622 (2023): 393–401.

24. Personal communication.

25. A. Joseph Tector, "Xenotransplantation in Humans: A Reality Check," *Transplantation* 109, no. 2 (2025): 231–234.

26. Roni Caryn Rabin, "Alabama Woman Receives Nation's Third Pig Kidney Transplant," *New York Times*, December 17, 2024.

27. Rob Stein, "Recipient of Pig Kidney Transplant Reaches a Milestone," *NPR*, January 30, 2025.

28. Rob Stein, "Pig Kidney Transplant Fails After Patient Rejection," NPR News, April 11, 2025, https://www.npr.org/sections/shots-health-news/2025/04/11/g-s1-59637/pig-kidney -transplant-rejection.

29. Shaun Chaiyabhat, "Man Who Survived One of Four Ever Pig Kidney Transplants, Throws First Pitch at Fenway Park," WCVB Boston, June 12, 2025, https://www.wcvb.com/article /man-who-survived-pig-kidney-transplant-throws-first-pitch-fenway-park/65040557.

30. Smriti Mallapaty, "First Pig-To-Human Liver Transplant Recipient 'Doing Very Well,'" *Nature*, May 31, 2024.

31. Deeptee Jain, "This Founder Is Getting Closer to Solving the Organ Shortage," *Forbes*, March 9, 2023.

32. Daniel Eisenson, "Consistent Survival in Consecutive Cases of Life-Supporting Porcine Kidney Xenotransplantation Using 10GE Source Pigs." *Nature Communications* 15, no. 1 (2024): 3361.

33. Martine Rothblatt, *Virtually Human: The Promise—and the Peril—of Digital Immortality* (St. Martin's Press, 2014).

34. "Forum: Locke and Sykes," *Nature Biotechnology* 41, Jayme Locke and Megan Sykes, January 18, 2023 (podcast).

Index